Forest Therapy - The Potential of the Forest for Your Health

Angela Schuh • Gisela Immich

Forest Therapy - The Potential of the Forest for Your Health

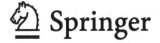 Springer

Angela Schuh
Chair of Public Health and Health Services
Research (IBE)
Pettenkofer School of Public Health
Ludwig Maximilians University
Munich, Germany

Gisela Immich
Chair of Public Health and Health Services
Research (IBE)
Pettenkofer School of Public Health
Ludwig Maximilians University
Munich, Germany

ISBN 978-3-662-64279-5   ISBN 978-3-662-64280-1   (eBook)
https://doi.org/10.1007/978-3-662-64280-1

Preface

More and more people are realising that living and spending their leisure time in the countryside is good for their health. The use of the forest as a place of rest, but also to do something for one's health, is becoming more and more important.

This non-fiction book *Forest Therapy—Potentials of the Forest for Your Health* (Waldtherapie—das Potenzial des Waldes für Ihre Gesundheit) aims to show the facts and background for the relevance of forest therapy in the context of our contemporary life on a scientific basis.

It is addressed to all those who are interested in the effects of nature and forests on human health and need well-founded information on this. Thus, those who want to do forest bathing themselves will get the necessary background knowledge. However, this book is also aimed at people in the health professions, psychologists and representatives of the "green professions", as well as doctors who deal with natural healing methods and those interested in learning more about the atmosphere of the forest and its health effects. In addition, this book provides a working basis for forest health trainers or forest therapists who want to instruct guests or patients in forest bathing or forest therapy on site.

We would like to thank the Springer staff, Ms. Monika Radecki and Ms. Anja-Raphaela Herzer, for the inspiration for this book and their professional, committed, and continuing support in the preparation of this book. The intensive discussions with both of them were a real enrichment. We would also like to thank Ms. Apurva Sarwade for her assistance with the English-language edition of our book.

Munich, Germany   Angela Schuh
August 2019   Gisela Immich

Contents

About the Authors

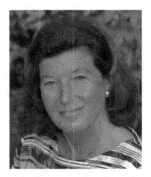

Angela Schuh Prof. Dr. rer. biol. hum., Dr. med. habil., Dipl. Meteorologist is Professor of Medical Climatology and Academic Director at the Chair of Public Health and Health Services Research (IBE) at Ludwig Maximilian University, Munich, Germany. She heads the Department of Medical Climatology, Health Resort Medicine and Prevention, and is an internationally recognised expert in climatotherapy and health resort medicine.

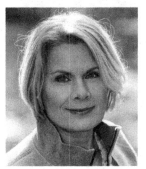

Gisela Immich, M.Sc., is a research associate at the Chair of Public Health and Health Services Research (IBE) at the Ludwig Maximilian University of Munich, Germany, and researches on the topics of forest therapy, health promotion and prevention as well as on various naturopathic healing methods.

List of Tables

1

Introduction

Summary

The topic of forests and forest therapy (forest bathing, Shinrin-Yoku) is on every-one's lips today. This corresponds to the new trend of "deceleration", which is due to our today's fast and often over-intensive life.

In our society, people hardly ever find relaxation. One is exposed to increasing and complex stresses resulting from both the working world and the personal social environment. Everything is happening faster and more concentrated. The job and often also the leisure life are characterized by hectic, stress and time pressure. Through IT technology, we are expected to be constantly available (day and night) and to react immediately. Even leisure life, which is characterized by activities, long-distance travel, fun sports, and thrills, no longer leaves time for rest, leaning back, reflection and relaxation. People have to react to these pressures and are often overwhelmed by them. Around eight out of ten Germans describe their lives as stressful, and one in three suffers from constant stress! Stress initially leads to mental and physical exhaustion, which is accompanied by a wide variety of functional disorders, e.g. in the cardiovascular system and sleep disorders. It is not without reason that psychological disorders such as burnout syndrome are among the most frequent reasons for sick leave. As a result of the constant exhaustion, chronic physical and mental illnesses develop.

So there is an urgent need for emotional, mental and physical balance! More and more people are realising that this can be achieved by spending

© Springer-Verlag GmbH Germany, part of Springer Nature 2022
A. Schuh, G. Immich, *Forest Therapy - The Potential of the Forest for Your Health*,
https://doi.org/10.1007/978-3-662-64280-1_1

time in nature, especially in the forest. The forest can be seen as a place for time out and as a source of strength and meaning—it is becoming a place of longing for many people in the context of modern life.

Forest therapy gives people a well-founded opportunity to do something for the health of body and mind, so far mainly in a preventive sense.

You can simply go to the forest and spend time there walking or resting. However, it can be assumed that the health-promoting effects are greater and more intense if you immerse yourself in the atmosphere of the forest with the help of special exercises and expose yourself to it in a targeted and well-dosed manner.

There are numerous studies on the preventive effects of the gentle forest climate, which show very clear mechanisms of effects. The health-promoting benefits of forest therapy for healthy individuals are undisputed. This is mainly shown by studies that have been carried out since the 1990s, mainly in Asia. Concerning the effects on existing diseases, the scientific findings are still relatively limited.

If one looks at the current literature on the subject of "forests and health", one quickly gets the impression that the forest is now the miracle cure par excellence. Often promises of healing are suggested, which are only conditionally or insufficiently confirmed by the scientific data.

Therefore, this book would like to contribute to summarise the scientific interrelationship and results in the field of forest and health for the layman understandably, to evaluate as well as to provide some, by investigations secured recommendations for the health-promoting use of the forest climate and forest therapy (forest bathing, Shinrin-Yoku).

2

Discovering the Forest: An Introduction

Summary

In this chapter, you will read about the important role the forest has always played in human life and how we can still use it today not only in its protective function and as an economic resource, but even as a place to maintain or improve our health. The importance of the forest and why the forest appeals to us is a good topic of our present time. It focuses on forest therapy, which can also be called Shinrin-Yoku or forest bathing.

With an area of 11.4 million hectares, one-third of Germany is forested and it is one of the most densely forested countries in the European Union (Bundesministerium für Ernährung und Landwirtschaft 2017). Of this, 51% is in public hands and 49% is owned by private individuals. In purely arithmetical terms, each German has 1300 m² of forest area at his or her disposal.

The forests consist of 90 billion old and young spruce, pine, beech, oak and rarer tree species. Today, spruce still dominates with 28% frequency, followed by pine with 23%, beech with 15% (declining) and oak, which has become rare today, with 10%. The share of deciduous trees is increasing again (Bundesministerium für Ernährung und Landwirtschaft 2017), the area ratio today is about 55% (conifers) to 45% (deciduous trees). Compared to other countries, only a few tree species are present in German forests, only 0.1% of the global diversity is found.

© Springer-Verlag GmbH Germany, part of Springer Nature 2022
A. Schuh, G. Immich, *Forest Therapy - The Potential of the Forest for Your Health*,
https://doi.org/10.1007/978-3-662-64280-1_2

2.1 Forest in the History of Human Development

A man originally comes from nature, he has lived in caves and forests and comes from green spaces. Unconsciously, one thus has an intuitive bond with nature stemming from evolution. Several theories deal with this. For example, the so-called biophilia hypothesis (see Sect. 2.2) states that all humans are designed by evolution to be in nature (Wilson 1984). Also, environments that have been shown early to be conducive to survival (food, safety), trigger positive responses and relaxation in humans (Ulrich 1993). In addition, natural scenery, i.e. landscapes are thought to be easily and effortlessly grasped and processed by humans (Bratman et al. 2012). All of this may provide a rationale for humans to be attracted to and comfortable in a natural environment. Thus, nature corresponds to human imprinting.

The forest plays a major role in our *evolutionary history.* There is much to suggest that human existence originated in forests. The first humans probably lived in forests and caves. In the course of cultural development, they then moved into huts, farms and villages. Only individual people retreated into the forests as so-called "hermits" (Keller 2018). For our ancestors, the forests were elementary, because in them they found shelter, raw materials such as wood as fuel and building material, and food in the form of animals and wild berries.

The forest has been experienced differently in the course of human cultural development from late antiquity to modern times (Keller 2018). In Germanic or Norse mythology, trees were worshipped as gods or attributed to them, e.g. the oak to the God Thor, the yew as the seat of the fertility goddess Rinda or the willow as the tree of the goddess of youth Iduna (Woelm 2006). The linden tree was used by the Germanic tribes as a court tree for the administration of justice, as it was believed to have divination and healing powers and to indicate the truth (Forstbotanischer Garten und Pflanzengeographisches Arboretum der Universität Göttingen 2019). A court of law could also be held under a linden tree—if the accused was found guilty, he was summarily hanged from the same. One of the most famous German court linden trees, as well as one of the oldest in Europe, is the 1200-year-old linden tree in Bad Staffelstein.

Hardly any of the tales or courtly novels from the High Middle Ages could do without the forest. In the Middle Ages, dark forests were perceived as threatening and people were afraid to go into the woods. Accordingly, in the Song of the Nibelungs, Siegfried was murdered by his adversary during a hunting trip under a linden tree in the forest. Many old trees were cut down with the onset of Christianity to eliminate the pagan idols. In the nineteenth century, the forest was experienced as particularly mystical. During the Romantic period, forests regained great importance in connection with the transfiguration of nature and longing for landscapes and were perceived as a place for living, recreation and retreat. Artists and painters dedicated their works to the forest. One of the most important musicians of the Romantic period, Felix Mendelssohn-Bartholdy (1809–1847), created his cycle of forest songs "Lieder im Freien zu singen" ("Sing songs outdoors"), a well-known example of which is the "Herbstlied" ("Autumn song"). Joseph Eichendorf (1788–1857) highlighted the forests in his poems such as "Abschied vom Walde" ("Farewell to the Forest"), and Caspar David Friedrich (1774–1840) immortalised the coastal forests of the Baltic Sea in his paintings. The "Ode an den Wald" ("Ode to the Forest", "Wandrers nightsong"), written by Goethe in 1776 after a walk in a gloomy spruce forest, also pioneered German Romanticism (Bundesministerium für Ernährung und Landwirtschaft 2018). The Brothers Grimm published their first fairy tale volume in 1812 with "Hänsel und Gretel" ("Hansel and Gretel"), one of the most famous fairy tales in which the deep forest is the setting. From this time on, almost all fairy tales are set in the forest—another very well-known example is "Rotkäppchen und der Wolf" ("Little Red Riding Hood and the Wolf") (Gustave Dore 1883). These descriptions still shape our image of the forest today.

During the German Third Reich, forests and the entire romanticism of the forest were glorified. This was reflected in the numerous forest scenes and forest theming (Keller 2018) in the music-dramatic works of Richard Wagner (1813–1883). During and after wartime, the forest continued to play a major role, as people now went into the forest to search for food. So spending time in the forest, whether walking or picking berries and mushrooms, became popular. In the years after the Second World War, the forest then became the setting for "perfect world" films such as "Geierwally" (1956) or "Förster vom Silberwald" ("forester of the silver forest") (1954). From this time onwards, the forest developed into a source of income for many people through forestry (according to the Bundesministerium für Ernährung und Landwirtschaft 2018), still today for 1.1 million people. In 1970, the first national park in Germany was founded.

In 1990, a forest was even the backdrop for a world-historical event, when Russian leader Michail Gorbatschow and the German Chancellor Helmut Kohl negotiated the terms of German reunification during walks in the forest. The photo of the two of them holding talks while sitting on tree stumps went around the world at the time (Bundesministerium für Ernährung und Landwirtschaft 2018).

However, in the 1980s and 1990s, there was the spectre of forest dieback, and forests became associated with the more troublesome issue. In the meantime, the forest was recovering, according to the Bundeswaldinventur des Bundesministeriums für Ernährung und Landwirtschaft (Bundesministerium für Ernährung und Landwirtschaft, Bundeswaldinventur 2019), which took place in 2011 and 2012. Today, however, climate change is putting new and existential stresses on the forest. Storms that produce increased wind breakage are on the rise, as heavy rain events and hot days or heat waves. For example, forests suffered greatly from heat, drought, hurricanes and bark beetle infestations during the long hot summer of 2018 and from snow breakage during the following severe winter of 2018/2019. As such weather conditions will occur more frequently in the future according to unanimous scientific findings, the forests will also be increasingly affected by them.

Situation Today

Since the 1960s, afforestation has been stepped up, and forest areas in Germany are increasing again by around 10,000 hectares per year (Scobel 2018). The protective function of forests continues to be elementary and often prevents landslides, floods and other natural disasters. Forests, together with the oceans, ensure that freshwater reservoirs are filled, the soil remains fertile and the climate has fewer extremes. Today, however, the forest is mainly considered from the point of view of environmental protection, but above all in connection with the timber industry. Thus, it is mainly about energy and material cycles. In addition, the forest is increasingly seen as a recreational area.

Many people, especially older people, still go into the forest frequently. They have already experienced from their grandparents and parents during extended Sunday walks in the forest how beautiful a stay in the forest is and how it benefits. They have retained this experience and, even as seniors, continue to seek out the forest in their free time. Keeping a dog supports this even more.

However, for younger people, especially those living in cities, spending time in the forest is often no longer an issue. In 1990, almost three-quarters of all local children still played outdoors; today, far fewer than half of them do so in industrialised nations (e.g. Brämer 2018a). Children live mainly indoors, spending more time in front of screens than outdoors. This is also confirmed by a German survey on the amount of time young people and adults up to the age of 29 use media (ARD and ZDF 2019). For example, the average media consumption in 1964 was about 210 min/day, whereas in 2015 an average of

560 min was spent in front of or with a digital device. That corresponds to about 9 h a day!

Spending hours in the forest is thus often a completely new experience for children and adolescents (Scobel 2018) and at most reminds them of "going for a walk in the forest with grandma". For young people, nature is rather unattractive, as new social contacts can hardly be created there (Dean et al. 2018). However, this "alienation from nature" is not only highly prevalent among children, but also middle-aged adults. In today's society, there has been a fundamental shift in values towards sedentary (indoor) activities with electronic media, which is accompanied by a reduced or non-existent appreciation of nature (Pergams and Zaradic 2006). Only people with a higher age still seem to value nature as a habitat with its biodiversity significantly more, as it can often be associated with personal memories.

Despite all this, the forest seems to be gaining in importance again. This is shown by a population survey, which found that nature is part of a good life for the German population and is associated with health and recreation (Bundesamt für Naturschutz 2012). An evaluation of various online sources (e.g. blogs, forums, etc.) also goes in this direction and indicates that nature has become more important to Germans. While the value of nature was still in fourth place in 2016, it has now secured the top position and was even judged more important than the value of health (Brämer 2018b).

2.2 Forest in the Context of Knowledge About Natural Areas

Natural environments contribute to recovery from emotional and cognitive exhaustion (Kaplan and Kaplan 1989). Nature offers ideal conditions for finding meaning and personality: Stimulating colours, shapes, smells and feelings allow people to distance themselves from everyday life and promote relaxation and well-being. This creates good conditions for better self-reflection (Ragettli et al. 2017). Spending time in nature has a positive effect on mood and concentration, creates contrasting experiences and enables stress reduction through comprehensive psychological and emotional relaxation (Bundesamt für Naturschutz 2018).

Theoretical Constructs
Spending time in nature has stronger positive effects on people than urban areas, this was already recognized by one of the founders of the so-called

ecopsychology (Wohlwill 1983). This field of research deals with the health-promoting aspects of human interactions with nature, and its representatives developed three theories for this purpose: The theory of stress reduction through natural landscapes, the attention-restoration theory, and the biophilia hypothesis.

The *theory of stress reduction* (Ulrich 1981) aims at the fact that the sight of a landscape results in immediate affection, i.e. non-volitionally controlled aversion. The recreational effect in nature begins within a very short time, i.e. within the first few minutes. Especially if an acute stress load has been experienced before, the sight of natural landscapes is said to have a clear stress-reducing effect. Even a simple, but much-cited experimental study with patients after a gall-bladder operation (Ulrich 1984) shows that healing was faster, the consumption of painkilling medication was lower and, in addition, the patients could be discharged 3 days earlier if they lay in a room with a view of the greenery—in contrast to those who looked at a wall opposite the window.

Almost all types of the landscape have a similar restorative effect on people (Ulrich et al. 1991), provided that no sense of insecurity or danger is conveyed, for example by highly unstructured or dense forest.

The *theory of attentional recovery* (Kaplan and Kaplan 1989) refers to effortless or unfocused attention to the complexity of landscape features as well as a certain fascination that comes from varied landscapes. This theory emphasises the importance of cognitive mechanisms. The basic assumption is that people have only a limited capacity or energy/time for directed attention; going beyond this can lead to mental exhaustion. If a mentally exhausted person then visits a natural landscape such as a forest, he comes to rest and strengthens his mental resources again, since nature does not demand directed, i.e. focused attention. Four basic cornerstones are said to be essential for this: The absence of daily stressors and problems/tasks, the feeling of emotional connection with nature and a certain fascination, which is exerted by the landscape so that automatically the attention falls voluntarily on it. These three factors are complemented by necessary compatibility between the person and their preferences for nature. The most important component is the aspect of the fascination of a landscape or nature. According to Kaplan's theory, the recovery process that takes place is described by four stages: First of all, "getting free of the head", in which the mental turmoil of thoughts becomes more and more silent. The second stage of relaxation describes the "recharging" of new unfocused, i.e. free attention. These first two stages lead to a calm state without being overwhelmed by a flood of thoughts. Now—and this represents phase 3—the person is again able to perceive his own ideas and thoughts. The fourth and deepest phase of relaxation then allows reflection on one's own life, the goals set, personal priorities, and the possibilities and opportunities that life could offer.

Nature thus provides a variety of different stimuli that enables mental recovery, as no prolonged focused attention performance needs to be maintained. Nature provides the feeling of "being away" from routine tasks and thoughts, and gently directs attention to brief interesting, even relaxing content without fixation.

The *biophilia hypothesis* (Wilson 1984) is based on the term of the same name, which was first developed by the psychoanalyst Erich Fromm in the 1930s (Becker 2009). This theory assumes that humans have an evolutionarily determined, genetically anchored need to approximate living beings as well as nature, not only physiologically and morphologically, but also in the form of certain social and psychological processes. Ultimately, this is to enable the survival of the human race in the earth ecosystem. However, this hypothesis is controversial because, on the contrary, man is also (justifiably) afraid, for example of wild animals, snakes or natural events.

Nature Stays
In addition to the theoretical concepts, emotional closeness to nature is also becoming more and more of a topic. *Connectedness to nature* has a health-promoting effect on mental and emotional health. It can reduce stress levels and increase overall well-being. There are links between lack of nature connectedness and various mental or psychological illnesses such as depression, anxiety and stress disorders (Dean et al. 2018).

People of all ages benefit from spending time in nature, because in addition to reducing stress, a natural environment increases physical activity (Kaczynski and Henderson 2007). For example, research shows that seniors in particular show an increase in coordination skills when they are regularly out in nature (Orr et al. 2016). Coordination is improved by walking on uneven paths. This has a positive effect in terms of reducing the risk of falls. Senior citizens basically like to go out in nature, because from their point of view it opens an opportunity for physical activity, but also sociability. They perceive nature in great detail, observe plant structures, the growth of plants or the change of seasons with the autumnal splendour of colour much more intensively and are happy about it. Perhaps contact with nature also contains a spiritual component: becoming one with nature and recognising the course of life, becoming and passing away and the return of life. Thus, a stay in nature is highly recommended for older people.

Even if mobility is already limited, seniors would like to enjoy nature more. For example, nursing home residents subjectively feel more comfortable when they live in a room with a view of the green (Orr et al. 2016). By having a view of greenery, they establish an individually strong connection to nature and enjoy or delight in it. This has a positive influence on subjective well-being.

Children's development is promoted by spending time in nature. The opportunities for free play and learning in nature sustainably promote children's cognitive, social and motor development. Spending time in nature thus lays the foundation for health awareness and well-being (Gebhard 2010). The various national forest education programmes promote visits to nature, contacts with nature and the knowledge and significance of these contacts.

Forests are natural areas and achieve a comparably high value as coastal areas in terms of recreation (White et al. 2013). Forest visits thus serve all aspects of closeness to nature. Experience shows that regular visits to woodlands at least 2 times per week can significantly enhance emotional connectedness to nature, whereas occasional visits to nature fail to maintain emotional connectedness (Clifford 2018).

In order to promote recreation in the German forest landscapes, the recreational function was amended to the German National Forest Act in 1973. In addition, the "recreational forest" was added to the Federal Forest Act in 1986, which serves day, weekend, holiday and spa recreation.

Forest Visit in Germany

In Germany, there are about 2 million forest visitors per year. Mountain bikers, hikers or walkers report almost exclusively positive experiences after visiting the forest (Arzberger et al. 2015). Scientists' surveys show that the varied sensory experiences in the forest have the greatest appeal for forest visitors (Schaffner and Suda 2008). The forest primarily serves as a recreational and adventure space for visitors to experience nature. The tranquillity, good air and fresh greenery are sensory impressions typical of forests that shape the memory of a visit to the forest and lead to rest, relaxation and well-being (Schaffner and Suda 2008; Arzberger et al. 2015). Another important reason to visit the forest for many people is to escape the hustle and bustle and confinement of the city (Shin et al. 2010). The forest can be seen as a "place of longing" for city dwellers who are tired of civilization (Nano 2017). However, the nature of forest use has been changing in recent years: although hiking and walking are still the most popular forms of recreation in the forest, sporting activities such as cycling, jogging and Nordic walking are increasing significantly (Lupp et al. 2017).

Forest visits with like-minded people can promote not only physical and psychological well-being but also social well-being (Nievergelt and Widrig 2008). They promote the experience of nature in the form of a sense of community and convey security and cohesion. Forest visitors unfamiliar with nature may therefore find it easier to open up to the unknown natural refuge if they are not alone or are guided. In urban green spaces, most people prefer to relax together (Staats and Hartig 2004).

Forest and Health

Enjoying the forest and exercising in the fresh air is good for human well-being. This has been known for a long time.

However, people go to the forests not only for recreation, but because they "may feel deep down that it serves their health" (Höppe and Mayer 1983).

After German scientists had already suggested at the end of the nineteenth century that forests could protect against cholera, research on the recreational function of forests and the use of the forest climate for recovery purposes has been carried out in Germany since the beginning of the twentieth century. A comprehensive description of the various phytoncides in the forest dates back as early as 1928 (Tokin and Kraack 1956).

The background to this was pulmonary tuberculosis prevalent at the time, which was treated by means of climatic therapy in the forest regions of the Harz or the Black Forest. The climatotherapeutic procedure "fresh air rest cure" (see Sect. 5.4.2) was described in the "Zauberberg" (Magic Mountain) (Mann 1991) as a treatment regime for pulmonary tuberculosis. At that time, there were a large number of pulmonary sanatoria in Germany's large forest areas, such as in the Harz mountains and Switzerland.

In Asia, too, the question of how forest areas promote or support health and recreational ability has been addressed since the early twentieth century. It is only in recent years that the wave of Shinrin-Yoku has "spilled over" from Asia to Central Europe, and spending time in the forest and its possible health effects are becoming more and more important.

2.3 What Is Forest Bathing/Forest Therapy?

"Forest bathing" is derived from the Japanese original "Shinrin-Yoku" (Lee et al. 2013). Shinrin-Yuko means "*immersion in the atmosphere of the forest*". Loosely translated, it is also often paraphrased as "forest bath" or "forest air bath". In Japan Shinrin-Yoku is also called "forest therapy" or "forest medicine". Here, "forest therapy" is defined as a programme in which forest bathing is undertaken for the maintenance of vitality and general mental health, as well as for the prevention of disease (Imai 2013).

The two German terms "Waldtherapie" (forest therapy) and "Waldbaden" (forest bathing) are not clearly separable. In the opinion of the authors of this book, the term "Waldbaden" should really only be applied to the stay of healthy people in the forest. "Forest therapy," on the other hand, includes therapeutic measures or interventions in the forest for existing medical conditions beyond health promotion and prevention. If patients are to be treated by means of forest therapy, then appropriately trained medical personnel are also required (see Sect. 5.2).

Shinrin-Yoku has a decades-long tradition in Japan and Korea. The term "Shinrin-Yoku" was first coined in 1982 by the head of Japan's Forestry Administration, Tomohide Akiyama (Miyazaki 2018). The birthplace of Shinrin-Yoku is considered to be the particularly aesthetic and mysterious Akasawa Forest in central Japan. Thus, the first forest therapy base was opened in the Akasawa Natural Recreational Forest in 2006, with the development of "Forest Stations" based on the Kneipp concept of health resorts in Germany (Kagawa 2019). There, stress-ridden Japanese can follow an individually tailored programme under the guidance of qualified forest therapists on eight Shinrin-Yoku trails of varying degrees of strenuousness. This is preceded by a medical "Forest Therapy Check-Up", where the visitor has prescribed a one-day or multi-day Shinrin-Yoku programme (Li 2018).

For the Japanese, Shinrin-Yoku is about finding peace, letting oneself drift and consciously perceiving the forest and its special conditions in order to regain strength for everyday life. Light walks or body-mind exercises such as Tai Chi are also incorporated. The whole population can participate in the guided forest bathing. But it has also become part of modern standard medicine in Japan as an additional service (3sat 2018; Scobel 2018). The International Society for Nature and Forest Medicine (INFOM) is focused on "forest medicine", but predominantly in the preventive sense (Li 2012).

Thus, more than 100 forest therapy centres are to be established throughout Japan, so that every stress-ridden Japanese will have easy access to the health-promoting Shinrin-Yoku. There are already 63 forest therapy centres in Japan. The centres are certified (including certified Shinrin-Yoku trails, trained therapists, medical facilities with testing of cardiovascular function or stress levels, healthy food, good transport links, adapted infrastructure) (Immich 2018). "According to Japanese understanding, forest therapy is the practice of health-promoting recreational activities in a forest environment, conducted under the supervision of medically trained personnel, which leads to a holistic increase in health and well-being and produces demonstrable relaxation effects" (Adamek 2018; Immich 2018). However, there are also Shinrin-Yoku programmes in which participants are physically active and, for example, perform logging work or saw wood (Uehara 2017).

In South Korea, lifespan health promotion is promoted and implemented as a governmental task in the form of "Forest Welfare" and "Forest Therapy" (Park 2018). Through various projects and programmes in the forest, such as forest kindergartens, active programmes for children, adolescents and young adults, or recreational programmes for professionals, parents and seniors, the common good is more socially promoted. Low-income people or people with disabilities are financially supported to enable them easy access to the different programmes in the forests.

Internationally, forest therapy is advanced by the American "Association of Nature and Forest Therapy ANFT". There, the focus of forest therapy is less on walking or simply relaxing in the forest, but rather on "immersion" in the forest. Forest therapy places its focus on "connecting with nature" (Clifford 2018). Mindfulness plays a special role here.

In Finland, France, Ireland, Luxembourg, Sweden, Austria and Italy (South Tyrol), forest recreation is also carried out—partly with state support. In Denmark, people with stress-related illnesses are treated in a therapeutic forest or a forest therapy garden. In Germany, the first therapeutic forest has been opened in Mecklenburg-Western Pomerania, which is primarily aimed at rehabilitation patients, the chronically ill and senior citizens, but is also open to the healthy population and guests. There are also signs of a intensive development towards forest therapy in the other federal states. However, different programmes are offered under different names.

The Shinrin-Yoku is guided in Japan and other countries by "Forest Therapy Guides" or "Forest Therapists" or similar. In Germany, there are numerous coaches of all kinds. However, in order to ensure appropriate and verifiable quality, this task will have to be carried out by specially trained professionals in the future (see Sect. 5.2).

According to the meaning of the word Shinrin-Yoku, "immersion in the forest atmosphere" includes first of all the special atmosphere, which consists to an important part of the special forest climate. Then there are the other elements of the forest, such as its aesthetics.

The forest atmosphere is absorbed by a man with all his *senses:*

- The eyes receive different light conditions, mostly twilight, and see the forest structures and different colours.

- The sense of smell perceives new impressions, e.g. the smell of wood and earth.
- You can hear rare sounds, such as birdsong, the rustling of leaves or the babbling of a brook.
- With the tactile sensors of the hands, new materials can be sensed (leaves, bark, etc.).
- The sense of taste is stimulated, for example, by tasting berries.

Addressing each of the five senses has numerous health-promoting, calming, physical and emotional effects (see Sect. 3.4).

In principle, it can be assumed (see also studies in Chap. 4) that spending time in the forest is *calming and relaxing*. The relaxing effect of the forest can be experienced by simply resting, meditating and body-mind practices such as Yoga or Qigong. In addition, the forest is an excellent motivator for physical activity, although this should be light during Shinrin-Yoku. Exercise, such as walking in the forest or hiking, is known to be relaxing and has many other health benefits. Therefore, the compliance for well-dosed and therapeutically guided climatic terrain treatment (see Sect. 5.4.2), hiking, gymnastics, Tai Chi exercises (see Sect. 5.4.1) in the forest is significantly higher than, for example, in an indoor gym.

However, the *condition of the forest* also plays a major role in the well-being of people spending time in the forest—irrespective of other effects—whereby spending time in a well-kept or managed forest has a more positive effect on well-being than in a decaying forest. Another important prerequisite for well-being is safety in the forests; this applies above all to urban parks and urban or near-urban forests.

Despite all the positive aspects of forests for human health, it is also important to pay attention to the "*health of the forests*". "Of course, it is important that people once again walk through the forest with open eyes and all their senses and better understand the beauty of this habitat," is one forester's credo (Schreder 2018). But he also unmistakably points out that trees are plant life forms that grow, reproduce and die. Moreover, the forest is the habitat of many animals. Therefore, one should never forget to respect the forest habitat with all its inhabitants.

References

3sat (2018) Wunderwerk Wald. Mediathek. http://www.3sat.de/page/?source=/nano/umwelt/191816/index.html. Accessed 19 Dec 2018

Adamek MH (2018) Im Wald sein. Optimum Medien & Service GmbH, München

ARD und ZDF (2019) Tägliches Zeitbudget für die Mediennutzung in Deutschland in ausgewählten Jahren von 1964 bis 2015 (in Minuten). In: Statista – das Statistik-Portal. https://de.statista.com/statistik/daten/studie/462835/umfrage/zeitbudget-fuer-mediennutzung-in-deutschland/. Accessed 19 Mar 2019

Arzberger M, Gaggermeier A, Suda M (2015) Der Wald: ein Wohlfühlraum. LWF aktuell 107:9–13

Becker M (2009) Wie zeitgemäß ist Biophilie? Erich Fromm und die Pädagogik der Postmoderne. https://www.fromm-gesellschaft.eu/images/pdf-Dateien/Becker_M_2009.pdf. Accessed 19 Mar 2019

Brämer R (2018a) Abschied von der Natur? Facetten einer schleichenden Naturentfremdung. Studien zur Natur-Beziehung in der Hyperzivilisation. https://www.natursoziologie.de/files/ne-recherche-02_1803241530.pdf. Accessed 19 Mar 2019

Brämer R (2018b) Werteindex Natur. https://www.natursoziologie.de/files/4-werteindex_1807291841.pdf. Accessed 19 Mar 2019

Bratman GN, Hamilton JP, Daily GC (2012) The impacts of nature experience on human cognitive function and mental health. Ann N Y Acad Sci 1249:118–136

Bundesamt für Naturschutz (2012) Erholung und Wohlbefinden. https://natgesis.bfn.de/fachwissen-gesundheit/gesundheitsfoerderung-und-praevention/erholung-wohlbefinden.html. Accessed 19 Mar 2019

Bundesamt für Naturschutz (2018). https://natgesis.bfn.de/fachwissen-gesundheit/gesundheitsfoerderung-und-praevention/erholung-wohlbefinden.html. Accessed 26 July 2018

Bundesministerium für Ernährung und Landwirtschaft (BMEL) (2017) Waldbericht der Bundesregierung 2017. Kurzbericht. https://www.bmel.de/SharedDocs/Downloads/Broschueren/Waldbericht2017Kurzfassung.pdf?__blob=publicationFile. Accessed 19 Mar 2019

Bundesministerium für Ernährung und Landwirtschaft (BMEL) (2018) Der Wald in der Weltgeschichte – eine Zeitreise durch unser Waldkulturerbe. Bonn. https://www.bmel.de/SharedDocs/Downloads/Broschueren/Waldkulturerbe-ZeitstrahlA4.pdf;jsessionid=4ECB75C26D57CBD9B4B9C7C764B62D41.1_cid288?__blob=publicationFile. Accessed 19 Aug 2018

Bundesministeriums für Ernährung und Landwirtschaft (BMEL) (2019) Dritte Bundeswaldinventur 2012. https://www.bundeswaldinventur.de/. Accessed 19 Mar 2019

Clifford A (2018) Your guide to forest bathing. Conari Press, Newburyport

Dean JH, Shanahan DF, Bush R, Gaston KJ, Lin BB, Barber E, Franco L, Fuller RA (2018) Is nature relatedness associated with better mental and physical health? Int J Environ Res Public Health 15:1371

Forstbotanischer Garten und Pflanzengeographisches Arboretum der Universität Göttingen (2019) Im Reich der Bäume – von Hexenhaar und Holzpantoffeln. http://www.uni-goettingen.de/de/im+reich+der+b%c3%a4ume/10235.html. Accessed 19 Mar 2019

Gebhard U (2010) Wie wirken Natur und Landschaft auf die Gesundheit, Wohlbefinden und Lebensqualität? In: Bundesamt für Naturschutz (Ed) Naturschutz & Gesundheit. Allianzen für mehr Lebensqualität, Bonn. https://www.bfn.de/fileadmin/MDB/documents/ina/vortraege/2011/2011-Naturbewusstsein-Gebhard.pdf. Accessed 20 Mar 2019

Höppe P, Mayer H (1983) Bioklimatische Aspekte des Waldklimas. Z Phys Med Balneol Med Klimatol 12:5–11

Imai M (2013) An introduction to the Forest therapy Society of Japan, Forest therapy® and Forest therapists®. In: Li Q (ed) Forest medicine. Nova Science Publishers, New York

Immich G (2018) Shinrin-yoku: symposium Waldmedizin. AFZ Wald 16:14–16

Kaczynski AT, Henderson KA (2007) Environmental correlates of physical activity: a review of evidence about parks and recreation. Leis Sci 29:315–354

Kagawa T (2019) Entwicklung der Forest Therapy Stations in Japan am Beispiel von Okutama. LMU Munich on Written message to Gisela Immich 15(02):2019

Kaplan R, Kaplan S (1989) The experience of nature. A psychological perspective. Cambridge University Press, New York

Keller HE (2018) Wagners Wälder – Beobachtungen zu Siegfrieds Waldleben. https://uni-salzburg.at/fileadmin/oracle_file_imports/1079186.PDF. Accessed 19 Mar 2019

Lee J, Park BJ, Tsunetsugu Y, Miyazaki Y (2013) Forests and human health – recent trends in Japan. In: Li Q (ed) Forest medicine. Nova Science Publishers, New York

Li Q (2012) Forest medicine. Nova Science Publishers, New York

Li Q (2018) Shinrin-yoku. The art and science of forest bathing. Penguin Life Random House, London

Lupp G, Förster B, Kantelberg V, Weber G, Pauleit S (2017) Stadtwald 2050. Endbericht. Lehrstuhl für Strategie und Management der Landschaftsentwicklung, Wissenschaftszentrum Weihenstephan, Technische Universität München

Mann T (1991) Der Zauberberg, 18. Aufl. Fischer Taschenbuch, Frankfurt

Miyazaki Y (2018) Shinrin yoku. Heilsames Waldbaden, Irisiana, München

Nano (2017) Wunderwelt Wald. Sendung vom 25.04.2017, 3Sat. http://www.3sat.de/mediathek/?mode=play&obj=66192. Accessed 20 Mar 2019

Nievergelt B, Widrig R (2008) Warum macht der Wald gesund? Runder Feldtisch in Bad Ragaz am 17. April 2008. Arbeitsgemeinschaft für den Wald, Schweiz

Orr N, Wagstaffe A, Briscoe S, Garside R (2016) How do older people describe their sensory experiences of the natural world? A systematic review of the qualitative evidence. BMC Geriatr 16:116

Park BJ (2018) Forest welfare policy in South Korea. Poster Präsentation am 2. Internationalen Kongress "Gesundheitspotential Wald" in Krems, Österreich vom 6.–7. November 2018

Pergams OR, Zaradic PA (2006) Is love of nature in the US becoming love of electronic media? 16-year downtrend in national park visits explained by watching movies, playing video games, internet use, and oil prices. J Environ Manag 80:387–393

Ragettli M, Flückiger B, Röösli M (2017) Auswirkungen der Umwelt auf die Gesundheit. Studie im Auftrag des Bundesamts für Umwelt der Schweizerischen Eidgenossenschaft. SWISS Tropical and Public Health Institute, Basel

Schaffner S, Suda M (2008) Erholungseinrichtungen im Urteil der Bürger – Sinnliches Naturerleben im Wald wichtiger als Wege, Hütten, Ruhebänke. LWF aktuell 62:12–15

Schreder T (2018) Zitat Lebensraum Wald. In: Förg N (Ed) Die Waldbademeisterin. Münchner Merkur extra vom 7. April 2018

Scobel G (2018) Patient Wald. Um unsere Wälder ist es schlecht bestellt. 3sat Scobel Wissensmagazin. http://www.3sat.de/scobel/190683/index.html. Accessed 31 Aug 2018

Shin WS, Yeoun PS, Yoo RW, Shin CB (2010) Forest experience and psychological health benefits: the state of the art and future prospect in Korea. Environ Health Prev Med 15:38–47

Staats H, Hartig T (2004) Alone or with a friend: a social context for psychological restoration and environmental preferences. J Environ Psychol 24:199–211

Tokin BP, Kraack E (1956) Phytonzide. Volk und Gesundheit, Berlin

Uehara I (2017) Therapy in forests in Japan. Lecture on the 1st International Congress "Health potential Forest" in the context of the opening of the 1st German cure and healing forests in Heringsdorf on the island of Usedom, Germany from 13.–14. September 2017

Ulrich RS (1981) Natural versus urban scenes: some psychophysiological effects. Environ Behav 13:523–556

Ulrich RS (1984) View through a window may influence recovery from surgery. Science 224:420–421

Ulrich RS (1993) Biophilia, biophobia, and natural landscapes. In: Kellert SR, Wilson EO (eds) The biophilia hypothesis. Island Press, Washington, DC

Ulrich RS, Simons RF, Losito BD, Fiorito E, Miles MA, Zelson M (1991) Stress recovery during exposure to natural and urban environments. J Environ Psychol 11:201–230

White MP, Alcock I, Wheeler BW, Depledge MH (2013) Coastal proximity, health and well-being: results from a longitudinal panel survey. Health Place 23:97–103

Wilson EO (1984) Biophilia. Harvard University Press, Cambridge

Woelm E (2006) Mythologie, Bedeutung und Wesen unserer Bäume. Monsenstein und Vannerdat, Münster

Wohlwill JF (1983) The concept of nature. In: Altman I, Wohlwill JF (eds) Human behavoir and environment. Springer, Plenum Press, New York

3

The Atmosphere: Forest Climate and Its Health Effects

Summary

Shinrin-Yoku describes "bathing in the atmosphere of the forest". This chapter is about the atmosphere of the forest. It is based on the special climatic factors of forests and their exchange with the environment and the overall atmosphere. We perceive and process the forest atmosphere with all our senses, which includes the structure of the forest and its aesthetics. All these individual elements of the forest atmosphere have concrete health-promoting or even therapeutic effects, which are also demonstrated.

3.1 Forest Climate

The climate inside the forest differs considerably from the open land. Forests have *their own local climate*, which can vary depending on the tree species, foliage, the height of the trees and density of the stand. In addition, the climatic conditions inside the forest are vertically graded and differentiated into the canopy, stem space and soil area. The canopy of a forest is the outer active surface with which it separates itself from the atmosphere; it regulates the exchange of energy and matter and leads to the formation of the special forest interior climate. The forest climate, which is relevant for the stay of humans in the forest, is located in the trunk area and on the forest floor.

The forest climate is predominantly beneficial to health and has a protective function against climatic or current weather influences as well as numerous environmental impacts. It is characterised by the following properties:

© Springer-Verlag GmbH Germany, part of Springer Nature 2022
A. Schuh, G. Immich, *Forest Therapy - The Potential of the Forest for Your Health*,
https://doi.org/10.1007/978-3-662-64280-1_3

- Protection from strong sunlight
- Protection from heat and cold, balanced temperature conditions
- Increased humidity
- Protection from precipitation
- Reduced wind speed
- "Green lung", oxygen production
- Protection against air pollution
- Gas exchange with the atmosphere through the emission of volatile organic compounds (BVOCs)

In a broader sense, the forest climate also includes

- Noise protection, noise attenuation
- Gentle light conditions, twilight
- "Aromatic" forest air
- Soft forest floor
- Forest Sounds

The factors of *forest climate* are in detail (Table 3.1):

Solar Radiation

The entry of solar radiation into the forest is determined by the tree species, the density of needles and leaves, as well as by the season and the position of the sun. In coniferous forests and during the vegetation phase of deciduous trees from spring to autumn, only little radiation reaches the trunk area during the day. In a dense deciduous forest, 15–20% of global radiation is reflected, 70–80% is absorbed, and only 5–10% penetrates to the ground in the trunk area (Mayer 2003; Trenkle 1989). In the native German coniferous forest, sunlight is shaded even more than in the deciduous forest. Thus, only 5% of the sunlight reaches the ground throughout the year in a dense spruce forest and even only 1% in a very dense spruce stand. The average light intensity in a forest of spruce, fir or pine is also significantly reduced and amounts to between 2% and a maximum of 20% on an annual average under a sunny, cloudless sky (Kimmins 2003).

Therefore, the forest protects in summer against high UV radiation as well as heat radiation of direct solar radiation. Protection against excessive radiation is particularly strong in the interior of the forest, stronger in coniferous forests than in deciduous forests, coniferous forests provide shade all year round. But also on north-exposed edges of forests one is protected against intense solar radiation.

Table 3.1 Elements of the forest climate and their health-promoting effects

Elements of the forest climate	Notes	Health-promoting effects
Solar radiation	Radiation intensity (infrared, visible light, UV) significantly reduced, especially in the ground area. Coniferous forest shields more than deciduous forest.	Radiation is reflected and absorbed at the crown, hardly any radiation penetrates. In winter: Radiation from the crown, hardly any radiation near the ground, thus less cooling. Winter deciduous forest less shading.	Protection against heat stress, light protection, skin protection.
Air temperature	Cooler than ambient during the day and summer, especially near the ground. Warmer in the coniferous forest in winter. No extreme values.	Due to low radiation intensity (see above) and evaporation. Evaporation canopy (interception), leaves and needles (transpiration), forest floor (evaporation). Strongest in beech forests. Balancing effect of forests during bad weather.	Protection against heat stress, protection against cold. Exception: Clearings.
Humidity	Always high, because leaves and needles give off water vapour.	Humidity in the afternoon about 5–10% higher. Higher in dense stands than in loose ones.	Sultriness is possible on very hot days.
Precipitation	Strongly reduced in the interior of the forest.	Complete protection in light rain. In heavier rain, protection is up to 40%. Protective effect: Interception + stem drainage + dripping portion	Rain cover, protection from cooling.
Wind	Greatly reduced in the forest.	In the interior of the forest almost no wind. Conifers provide stronger wind protection than deciduous trees.	Wind protection, protection against cooling.

(continued)

Table 3.1 (continued)

Elements of the forest climate		Notes	Health-promoting effects
Gas exchange with the atmosphere			
Oxygen production	Rather insignificant.	Compared to the O_2 content of the atmosphere subordinate.	"Green lung"
Reduced or no air pollution/filtering effect	Filtering mainly of solid air impurities (particles, especially dust). Gases are filtered less.	High air purity inside a forest, but high ozone levels are possible in deciduous forests on very hot summer days.	Relief of the respiratory tract.
BVOC	Terpene and isoprene emission from coniferous and deciduous trees.	Heat promotes emission of terpenes in coniferous forests and isoprene in deciduous forests. Ozone reduction by BVOCs. But deciduous trees can in turn produce ozone precursors.	Still unclear.
Indirect forest climate factors			
Quietness	Noise significantly reduced.	Coniferous forests dampen particularly high frequencies, younger stands are more sound-absorbent	Noise control.
Twilight	Light intensity reduced	Especially inside the forest and near the ground. Also light plays and change of light/shadow. Green colour: Positive mood.	Calming, relaxing. Mental stimulation.
Forest air	Essential oils, resins and aromatic substances, mainly terpenes (conifers) responsible for odour	"Typical forest odour". Increased emission of terpenes at warm temperatures and after rain	Pleasant smell, connection to emotions.
Forest sounds	Diversity of sounds depending on species richness	Sun position and wind dependent: daylight=movement and sound; less sounds in winter	Emotional and psychological impact.
Forest floor	Soft and varied	Different walking requirements	Gentle on the joints and promotes coordination.

Air Temperature

If you go from the open air into a forest on a hot summer's day, you suddenly feel the coolness. In good weather conditions, the air in the open air warms up quickly after sunrise as a result of the sun's rays, whereas inside the forest it initially remains *cool and damp* for a longer period. The cool air in the forest is mainly due to the fact that only little direct solar radiation can penetrate the forest (see above). Pine stands—because they are sparser—have somewhat higher temperatures than spruce or deciduous forests (Flemming 1990).

The canopy warms up first. In densely leafy stands, the warming from the canopy to the forest floor continues slowly but steadily. The daily maximum temperatures in coniferous and deciduous forests in summer are therefore 4–5 degrees below those in the open land.

The lower temperatures of the forest interior climate in summer are—apart from the fact that only a small amount of radiation reaches the trunk area— also a consequence of the strong *evaporation*. The total evaporation of the forest is composed of the evaporation of the canopy (interception), the leaves and needles (transpiration) and the forest floor (evaporation). The forest releases about 70% of the received precipitation back into the atmosphere (Meyers Lexikon 1989). Because of the large vegetation surface, about 15–25% more precipitation evaporates in the forest than on agricultural land. On a summer day, a hectare of beech forest with about 100 trees can evaporate more than 50,000 L of water (which corresponds to about 330 filled bathtubs—an average bathtub holds 150 L). This is particularly noticeable on hot days. Since a lot of radiant energy is used for evaporation, which leads to cooling, it is significantly cooler inside a forest than in the surrounding area. Together with the already lower radiation intensity inside the forest, evaporation explains why the forest climate is several degrees cooler and more humid than the climate in the surrounding area during the summer season.

Among deciduous forests, beech forests in particular offer this significant temperature reduction. In terms of evaporation, deciduous and coniferous forests do not differ. A study in a forest near Vienna, Austria (Cervinka et al. 2014) showed that on hot summer days, a mixed stand of beech and spruce, which had four different tree heights (layers) and canopy areas of approximately 75%, already made the heat significantly more bearable and the test subjects felt that this stand was conducive to recreation. The shielding provided by the tree canopy plays a prominent role, with 100% canopy being the most suitable for coping with heat (Cervinka et al. 2014).

At night and in winter, the forest only slowly releases the heat stored during the day or in summer. Therefore, on cold winter days, it is *warmer* in the coniferous forest than in the surrounding area. On average, the air temperature in winter is about 1 degree above the outdoor temperature. In the deciduous forest, there is a strong cooling after the loss of leaves, with almost unimpeded rain and snow and unhindered penetration of solar radiation, similar to that in the open air.

In bad weather, the *balancing effect* of forests is particularly noticeable (Trenkle 1989). Large temperature fluctuations are mitigated, as well as violent winds and strong gusts of wind (see below).

In forest clearings, more solar radiation can penetrate, and there the summer warming continues more quickly until close to the ground. However, ventilation is less than in the open. Therefore, during summer high-pressure periods, forest clearings or thinned stands can become significantly warmer during the day and significantly cooler at night than in the surrounding area (Trenkle 1989).

Humidity

The relative humidity in the forest is 5–10% higher than in the lowlands due to the low air movement and the evaporation surfaces effective in the canopy and on the forest floor (see above) (Trenkle 1989). In a comparison with a nearby large city, values in the trunk area of a spruce forest were found to be up to 25% higher in summer.

The water vapour pressure, i.e. the actual amount of water vapour in the air, is higher in dense stands than in loose ones. During the day, the vapour pressure increases and reaches its maximum value of about 1 hPa in the afternoon (Flemming 1990). This causes an increase in relative humidity in the forest of about 5–10%. Therefore, relative humidity can be higher in forests in summer than in the open air (Höppe and Mayer 1983). On cloudy, warm summer days with little radiation, it can become sultry in the forest due to the lack of wind and the higher humidity.

During fog, the forest "combs out" large amounts of fog precipitation (droplets deposited from fog), especially at the stand edges. I.e. the pollutants present as condensation nuclei in the fog droplets and those dissolved in them due to the usually larger surface area of the fog droplet are then absorbed into the leaf and can be stored there. In winter, fog-frost deposits on the trees can paint bizarre pictures and particularly aesthetic forest impressions.

Rain

In the case of only light and short-lasting precipitation, the crown area completely shields the rain (Höppe and Mayer 1983). Each tree species protects differently from precipitation. To determine how strongly the crowns keep out the rain, the "crown wetting degree", up to which no drop falls to the ground, was defined. Thus, in conifers, 2–3 mm of rain is kept out in the crown area, and no drop falls to the ground. In a deciduous forest, one is completely protected from a rainfall of 1 mm.

Even in the case of heavier rainfall above the crown wetting level, the trees still reduce the amount of water considerably by a certain proportion of the precipitation already evaporating from the leaves or needles in the crown area and thus not reaching the ground at all. This process, known as interception, can amount to 20–30% of the rain in spruces and about 10% in beeches.

In addition, part of the precipitation—in the order of 10–30%—flows from the crown along the branches to the trunk and down the trunk to the ground. Trunk runoff depends on the roughness of the trunk. In the case of beech, stem runoff can amount to 15% of precipitation, and in the case of spruce, about 10%.

The precipitation in the forest is thus composed of three components: The interception, the stem flow and the dripping component.

Temporary adhesion of water can occur on the leaves. This happens due to the "splash", the bursting of raindrops on the leaves or the formation of giant drops, where many small droplets unite. Therefore, standing under a deciduous tree, one can also be hit by large and heavy drops. To summarise, humans are completely protected in the forest during weak rainfall and are only exposed to up to 40% less intensity during heavier rainfall.

Wind

Forests reduce wind speed mainly in the trunk area.

When the wind hits the forest and it is obstructed by dense vegetation, it must rise on the windward side, flow over the forest and sink again on the back side, i.e. in the lee (Fig. 3.1).

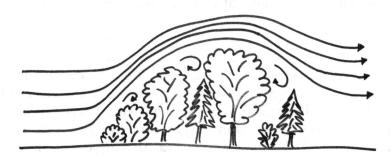

Fig. 3.1 Wind flow path over the forest (Immich 2019)

In the crown area the wind pressure acts, the forest begins to rustle ("forest rustle "). In strong winds, the crowns bend in the wind, there are swirls and turbulence, which can sometimes lead the wind into somewhat deeper layers of the forest. Horizontally, the wind does not penetrate very deep into the forest. At wind speeds of around 3 m/s, after 4 m there is only a speed of 1 m/s inside the forest (Trenkle 1989). From then on there is almost no wind. In clearings, however, turbulences occur which originate from the canopy. If glades run in the main wind direction, a jet effect with wind breakage can occur at high wind speeds. Even if the approaching wind is very turbulent, there is an exchange-related coupling of the air inside the forest with the outside air. Thus spatial wind differences are compensated, wind also blows in the forest and the windbreak function is at least reduced. In the lowlands, the windbreak effect of the forest (Flemming 1990) is stronger than in hilly areas.

Coniferous forests have the strongest protective effect due to the fine structure of the dense needles. They also provide year-round wind protection. This is an important effect, especially in coastal forests. Deciduous forests also provide good wind protection. The protective effect of both types of forest is better the denser the stand and with low-hanging branches. Surprisingly, the bare branches and trees of a winter deciduous forest still have half the windbreak effect as in the leafy state, i.e. still relatively much (Flemming 1990).

At the forest edges facing away from the wind, a transitional climate with lower wind speeds is found. This is due to the upward flow of air on the side facing the forest and the downward flow of air on the side away from the wind (lee). This affects a horizontal area of about 1.5 times the stand height at the forest edges. After the overflow, for example, of a dense fir stand, the wind speed on the lee side (side facing away from the wind) is reduced by 70–80% compared to the open land.

Sometimes a so-called forest wind develops at the edges of the forest. It is a balancing current between the cooler interior of the forest and the warmer surrounding area and flows out of the forest to the outside. However, its effectiveness usually extends only 20–60 m (Trenkle 1989).

Oxygen

Forests are often referred to as "green lungs". This term derives from the fact that, in purely mathematical terms, the gross production of oxygen from about five individually standing large trees or 20 forest trees in an old-growth stand corresponds to the daily oxygen requirement of a human being (Baumgartner 1977/78). However, since the oxygen supply from the atmosphere is completely sufficient and humans cannot intake anymore, this is a purely theoretical consideration that plays no role in "real life", but which has coined the term "green lung".

It is a fact (Mayer 1986) that every gram of assimilated carbon dioxide is matched by the release of 0.73 g of oxygen. If, however, the net assimilation is based on the respiration of trees (which takes place at night and during which O_2 is absorbed and CO_2 is released), it becomes apparent that the oxygen production of trees plays only a subordinate role for humans because of the relatively large atmospheric supply of O_2. Much more important is the storage effect of carbon dioxide in the leaves and trunk, which is elementary for our environment in the context of climate change.

Clean Air

Extensive forest areas represent a large reservoir of clean air, because the trees consume carbon dioxide and produce oxygen. In addition, the leaves and needles of the trees filter anthropogenic pollutants such as solid particles of different sizes (soot and dust particles) or gaseous admixtures out of the air. A healthy hundred-year-old tree can filter about 1 ton of air pollutants per year. The *filtering effect* depends in particular on the leaf surface. Using computer simulations, it was calculated that trees and forests in Canada filtered around 17.4 million tonnes of air pollutants from the atmosphere in 2010 (Nowak et al. 2014). In a European comparison, Douglas fir and spruce as well as beech and oak show a high uptake capacity for air pollutants due to their large leaf area index (Smidt 1999). In this context, 1 hectare of spruce stand can filter more dust from the air by a factor of 1.5 than a pure beech forest (Smidt 1999).

Air pollutants occur in solid, liquid and gaseous consistencies: The solid particles—the aerosol—have particle sizes ranging from submicroscopic to the millimetre range. In their capacity as pollutants, aerosol particles are divided according to size into respirable, breathable particles (fine dust) and non-breathable particles (coarse dust). Respirable particles are smaller than about 10 μm and consist mainly of combustion products such as soot and substances contained in fuels such as heavy metals and sulphur compounds. Fine dust with even smaller particle sizes poses a particular problem in this respect (see below). Coarse dust particles are produced by road abrasion among others, but they also include pollen and mite excrement. Gaseous air pollutants consist mainly of nitrogen dioxide, carbon dioxide and their reaction products such as ozone.

Especially for *solid particles*, also known as aerosols, forests are excellent filters. This is, where the large surface roughness of forests has an effect. How strong this filter effect will be, is depending on particle size as well as air movement.

When wind, with which the particles are transported, hits the forest, it can hardly penetrate the forest (see below), but must practically flow over the forest. The smaller a particle and the greater the wind speed, the more precisely the particles follow the streamlines of the air movement. During this process, they are lifted upwind by the forests and swirled around above them because of the great roughness of the crowns. On the leeward side of the forests, the particles then sink to the ground with the air movement. When there is strong air movement/wind, the filtering effect by the forest is greatest.

However, if the air movement is lower, this effect is weaker and the particles sink more into the forest. Then the particles are initially deposited in the crown area. Particles can also be transported to the forest from the surrounding area when there is only very slight air movement or barely noticeable wind. Then they cannot be carried beyond the crowns at all, but penetrate directly into the forest edge and are deposited on leaves, needles and twigs, as these hold the particles due to their great roughness. Thus, high concentrations of pollutants can accumulate at forest edges, with the horizontal deposition rate decreasing exponentially in the forest (Beier and Gundersen 1989). Spruce stands are particularly effective at filtering pollutants because of the large number of their fine needles and the resulting large surface area. Uneven, hairy leaves such as those of willow and hazel are better dust traps than smooth leaves. It can therefore be assumed that dense forests, especially those with low-hanging branches, have a very good filtering effect against air pollution.

When it rains, the particles deposited on the canopy and lower-lying leaves enter the trunk area or the air with the rainwater (see above).

Therefore, when it rains, a surprising situation can arise that the concentration of particulate matter in the precipitation in the area of the trunk—and thus the area where people are staying—is greater than outside the forest. The resulting air pollution is, however, wide-ranging in terms of magnitude. Thus, when it rains, the forest air can still be contaminated with particles due to the interception described above and the proportion that drips through. The particles from the canopy also reach the soil with the rain or later with leaf fall, to which trace substances are also increasingly added.

In the air of the forest interior, the concentration of solid particles decreases from above to the trunk area. The better air quality of the forest interior also continues in a relatively narrow marginal strip leeward of the forest. Therefore, trees and forests can make an important contribution to air purity concerning particulate pollutants, e.g. in cities (Nowak et al. 2018).

The protective effect against *gaseous pollutants* such as nitrogen oxides, sulphur dioxide, ammonia and carbon dioxide is, however—contrary to popular opinion—by far not as pronounced as for particles and is rather insignificant. The absorption capacity of plants for gases has been demonstrated but is limited. The relatively small proportion of gases that do not simply flow through forests (Jim and Chen 2008), but also experience a filtering effect, are mainly taken up via the leaves and absorbed on the surfaces of the plants. This results in damage to the leaves and needles. Due to the direct influence on cell metabolism, they discolour (turn yellow or brown) and die. Their resistance to frost and pests is also reduced (Moll 2013).

More than by the plant itself, the gases are absorbed by rainwater adhering to it. If the gaseous pollutants are dissolved in water (rain, fog), they enter the forest stand more directly. This applies in particular to nitrogen dioxide (NO_2). In the atmosphere, nitrogen dioxide reacts to nitrous acid and nitric acid, which leads to acidification of precipitation. As a result, NO_2 is deposited in the soil in the form of nitrate compounds. Due to their larger surface area compared to raindrops, fog droplets carry higher amounts of air pollutants and also bind pollutants in the form of condensation nuclei. Conifers "comb" air pollutants with their needles to a much greater extent than deciduous trees from moist air, as they have a larger leaf surface and retain their needles all year round (Bayerisches Landesamt für Umweltschutz 2015). In mountain forests (from about 1300 m altitude), this is particularly relevant, as a significant proportion (40%) of the total precipitation is caused by fog condensation (Pfadenhauer 1973).

About air purity in terms of gaseous pollutants, the components of isoprene and terpenes or terpenoids emitted by forests (see below) are gaining more and more scientific interest. Gaseous pollutants such as NO_2 can therefore be degraded by binding them to the BVOCs (see below).

At night and in the morning, the forest air contains a relatively high level of carbon dioxide. It originates from the respiration processes of the trees and the soil. Because the canopy weakens the vertical transport of CO_2 upwards, the values can exceed those of the surrounding area. During the morning, and especially when there is air movement, the situation quickly returns to normal. The diurnal differences in ozone depletion are similar: during the day, more ozone is depleted in the forest (see below); at night, when there is no wind, ozone levels can rise again.

Overall, the forest air is excellently protected, especially with regard to air pollution by solid particles such as fine dust, coarse dust, or soot through the stand surface and needles and leaves, and is thus significantly cleaner than the air of the surrounding area. For example, forests have an annual filtering effect of about 60 tons of dust per hectare (Moll 2013). This is even more significant today because virtually the entire environment—even outside cities—is polluted by fine dust. Due to its very small particle size, fine dust is transported many kilometres away from its point of origin. It is inhaled very deep into the lungs which are harmful to health (see Sect. 3.4). Only when it rains, forest air is charged with a higher level of fine dust due to the wash-off effect from the canopy. In principle, however, the air in the forest can be expected to be relatively low in particulate matter. The filtering capacity of the forest is significantly greater for solid and liquid particles than for gases.

Finally, forests assume a kind of "placeholder function" concerning gaseous and particulate pollutants (Höppe and Mayer 1983) and thus prevent the presence of emitters.

Gas Exchange with the Atmosphere

The exchange of gases between the tree and the atmosphere takes place through the stomata in the leaves. The tree breathes through them. This exchange is mainly controlled by the water vapour, the CO_2 concentration and the biochemical activity in the leaves or needles.

According to the latest scientific studies, the focus here is on volatile organic carbon compounds of plant origin (biogenic volatile organic components, BVOCs). These are a large number of different chemical compounds of natural origin, e.g. hydrocarbons, alcohols, aldehydes and organic acids. Their concentrations vary widely (ppt to ppb), their lifetimes range from minutes to hours, and some of them exhibit high chemical reactivity (Zemankova and Brechler 2010).

In Europe, forests emit the most BVOCs, while emissions from meadows play almost no role (Steinbrecher et al. 2009). Each forest produces its own site-specific mixture of BVOCs (Smiatek and Steinbrecher 2006).

The most common BVOCs emitted by plants and thus also by trees are isoprene and terpenes or terpenoids, also known as phytoncides (see below). They are chemically very reactive. Forests are the main sources of biogenic BVOC emissions. The emission is highly variable from tree species to tree species and even within the same species and is modified by environmental factors. Two comprehensive inventories of BVOC-emitting plant species and their excretion levels can be found at:

- www.es.lancs.ac.uk/cnhgroup/download.html of the biosphere-atmosphere Interactions and Atmospheric chemistry Research Group, Department of Environmental Science, Lancaster University, UK (Hewitt et al. 1997).
- https://doi.org/10.1007/978-1-4020-2167-1_4   by   Wiedinmyer et al. (2004).

Isoprene is synthesised in the stomata of the leaves of deciduous trees. Conifers, on the other hand, produce mainly terpenes and terpenoids. Few tree species emit both (Steinbrecher et al. 1997): The only representative of isoprene-emitting conifers in Germany is the common spruce. Among deciduous trees, considerably more species also emit terpenes. These include the silver poplar, some oak species such as red oak, pedunculate oak or downy oak, the robinia, the willow tree, the rotten oak, or the amber tree. In addition to trees, small plants can also emit isoprene and terpenes, for example, autumn daphne, broom and rush, heather, juniper or myrtle (Steinbrecher et al. 1997). Isoprene is the most widespread component—its annual emission is about half of the global BVOC emissions and is comparable to the total methane emission from all possible sources (Guenther et al. 2006; Sharkey et al. 2008).

Emissions of BVOCs, especially isoprene, are influenced by many meteorological factors. In principle, they are strongly dependent on the type of forest, season, daytime and nighttime temperature, leaf temperature, the brightness of daylight and sun position, as well as air humidity and wind speed (Smiatek and Steinbrecher 2006). Thus, in summer, outflowed BVOCs can increase abruptly at midday. During the leaf phase of deciduous trees in summer, the highest BVOC emissions are found in Europe: From June to August, deciduous forests produce more than 40% of the total annual amount of isoprene (Steinbrecher et al. 2009). The temperature dependence of BVOC emissions is shown, among other things, by the fact that in southern Europe BVOC emissions are higher than in northern Europe by a factor of 3 (Steinbrecher et al. 2009). Isoprene formation is not only influenced by air temperature, but also by the brightness of daylight (Rasmussen and Jones 1973). And the more direct the solar radiation (UVB) hits the leaves, the more is formed. When the sky is cloudy, isoprene production decreases again somewhat. The strength of isoprene emission is also controlled by leaf density and is thus additionally particularly seasonal (Zemankova and Brechler 2010). Deciduous trees in northern Europe, therefore, emit the most isoprene between May and September, but only 50% of the maximum value is reached in October and April. In the winter months between November and March, when deciduous trees no longer have any biomass available after leaf fall and when air temperature and daylight brightness are also low, they no longer produce isoprene.

This is different for conifers, which retain their needles throughout the year. In Germany, the large spruce stands account for the majority of BVOC emissions, at about 40% (Guenther 1997). They emit *terpenes and terpenoids* relatively constant throughout the year, controlled only by air temperature (Zemankova and Brechler 2010) and humidity. Thus, the composition of the "terpene cocktail" (of terpenes and numerous terpenoids) of coniferous forests is modified by air temperature (Kim 2001). In spring, when trees produce new fresh shoots/needles during the growing season, terpene concentrations are higher than in the rest of the year and the odour is altered (Cheng et al. 2009).

High humidity seems to increase the terpenes in the forest by about 70–80% (Lamb et al. 1993). This increased excretion of terpenes could explain why the forest smells very typically and intensively of "forest" or forest aromas (see below) after a rain shower. If it rains for 3 days in a row, the terpene content in the forest air increases by a factor of ten. In contrast, significantly fewer terpenes are emitted when the humidity is below 40%, for example in a sparse stand of trees during a summer drought.

The emission of BVOCs does not only depend on meteorological variables such as air temperature or humidity but is also increased by *stress* for the trees. This includes drought, for example, where there appears to be a complex relationship between air temperature, which increases terpene emission, and groundwater availability, which is the limiting factor in this. In deciduous trees, isoprene arguably provides effective protection against heat stress, as evaporation of isoprene from the leaf results in leaf cooling. As a result, deciduous trees have developed a protective mechanism that persists even when photosynthesis is no longer occurring due to reduced water supply (Lluisa et al. 2016). Thus, deciduous trees seem to cope better with high daytime temperatures than conifers. Other stressors for trees include attacks by predators, infestations by insects, microorganisms, or pathogens, which can lead to increases in BVOC emissions of up to 150% (Smiatek and Steinbrecher 2006). Movement or mechanical damage/breakdown also affects trees. Different authors also describe a 10- to 50-fold increase in the release of BVOCs when trees are exposed to stress from high winds or lightning (Juuti et al. 1990). Even mechanical touch seems to have an effect. Kim (2001) documented a 5- to 20-fold increase in emission of terpenes when touching branches/needles of loblolly pines (Pinus taeda). In addition to mechanical stress factors, age of the tree also affect the formation of BVOCs. Younger trees emit significantly more BVOCs than older ones.

BVOCs *interact with ozone*: the leaves and needles of trees, for example, absorb ozone from the ambient air, along with other air pollutants, by penetrating the stomata, where it causes considerable damage to the plant. Deciduous trees produce isoprene to prevent ozone damage. To a much lesser extent (see below), conifers produce monoterpenes that act as a kind of protective shield against ozone.

Especially the BVOC isoprene is an ozone precursors. It can form reactive oxygen radicals, which in turn can lead to the formation of ozone. Therefore, deciduous forests produce ozone on hot summer days (Wagner and Kuttler 2012). In cities with a high nitrogen dioxide concentration, on the one hand, increased ground-level ozone is formed by car exhaust gases; on the other hand, the newly formed urban smog ozone is immediately neutralised again by the inner-city greenery (trees).

Thus, in cities with heavy motor vehicle traffic, trees affect the neutralization or filtering of O_3 and particulate matter. If one balances the formation and reduction of ozone by BVOCs, it is quite clear that more ozone is depleted than newly formed (Nowak and Crane 2000). In particular, conifers, that emit little isoprene, can reduce O_3 pollution in cities.

In uncontaminated regions, isoprene will dilute the long-haul ozone that is transported away from the formation areas (Ibrahim et al. 2010).

The effects of pollutants on the biochemical response and the necessary conditions for trees that lead to BVOC emissions are still far from being conclusively understood (Calfapietra et al. 2013).

As forests absorb air pollutants more effectively than other forms of vegetation due to their large crown surface, they are also more severely affected by pollutants. Since the early 1980s, pines, beeches and oaks, in particular, have shown considerable damage. Despite measurable relief of forests from airborne pollutants, the crown condition of conifers has improved only slightly, except for spruces or pines (Bundesamt für Ernährung und Landwirtschaft 2017). In contrast, deciduous trees in Germany are doing increasingly worse. This can be observed in defoliation, i.e. thinning of the crowns. This damage occurs in all tree species, especially in older trees. The summer of 2018 was particularly damaging for the German forests. The extreme drought, a hurricane and an immense bark beetle infestation have destroyed entire sections of forest. German spruce stands in particular suffered from this (Nordrhein-westfälisches Ministerium für Umwelt, Landwirtschaft, Kultur- und Verbraucherschutz 2019).

Trees directly take up pollutants through the air, via the roots from the groundwater or the rainwater. The dust particles from the air adhere on the leaves or needles and fall to the ground or are washed off by rainwater. Gases can be absorbed particularly well (see above) when the leaves are moist and the gases can dissolve in the rainwater ("acid rain"): In Summer, sulphur dioxide and the nitrogen oxides in the air reach higher layers of air through air freights and updrafts. The air humidity condenses on them during rain formation, the pollutants dissolve in the rainwater and form sulphurous or nitrous acid. The rainwater thus becomes acidic and rains down on the ground as acid rain. In the soil, the input of the acid, even at low concentrations over a long period, leads to gradual acidification. As a result, the pH value in the groundwater and the water bodies decreases. The acid rain and also the ozone (which is filtered or chemically altered directly at the crown) additionally destroy the wax layer and the stomata of leaves and needles, which normally protect the leaves from drying out or regulate the water balance of the plant. As a result, the stomata can no longer close when it is too hot, and too much water evaporates. This additional missing wax layer causes much higher water evaporation. Due to the already damaged roots, the tree can no longer regulate its water balance and dries out.

Thanks to various air pollution control measures to reduce the emissions of acidic components through filtering systems or lower-sulfur fuels, our forests are doing considerably better in this respect—acidic inputs from rain are almost completely a phenomenon of the past (Dietrich et al. 2018). Instead, forest soils are increasingly under renewed pressure from excess nitrogen surplus from agriculture, high concentrations of ground-level ozone and negative impacts of climate change (Smidt 2004).

Quietness

In the forest, it is usually quieter than in the surrounding area or the open land. Forests have sound-absorbing properties due to the leaves, needles and branches of trees, shrubs and small plants. Two effects come into play here: Firstly, sound waves that propagate in the forest lose part of their energy when they hit the leaves because they are dispersed and reflected diffusely. Secondly, the sound waves cause the leaves to move, which results in the sound waves being further weakened in energy and altered in frequency. The soft forest floor also attenuates sound propagation (Ziemann et al. 2016). These effects were demonstrated many years ago (Mitscherlich and Schölzke 1977): Compared to a meadow, stands of oak trees attenuate sound by 15 decibel (dB) in summer, at a distance of 50 m from the noise source; a beech forests silencing noise by 13 dB, a spruce stand by 12 dB and a pine stand by

10 dB. Recent measurements also found that a 100 m wide, dense mixed forest with a densely stepped forest edge results in a sound reduction of 17–25 dB (Hehn et al. 2016). The attenuation effect can be effective in the forest up to 200 m behind the forest edge. Meteorological factors such as wind—especially headwind—and higher air temperatures also reduce sound propagation.

The sound attenuation also depends on the frequency. Thus, the greatest effect occurs at frequencies around 250 Hz, i.e. low sounds, and at 2000–4000 Hz, i.e. high sounds. A maximum sound reduction of 33 dB per 100 m horizontal distance from the sound source can occur. Sound attenuation is probably lowest around 500 Hz and in the middle range around 1000 Hz (Mayer 1986).

Coniferous forests such as spruce, fir and Douglas fir primarily attenuate sound waves with high frequencies. This is made possible by the fine structure of the needles, which strongly scatter or absorb the high-frequency sound waves and thus remove the energy from them again. This is a particularly important effect of coniferous forests because people perceive sound waves with high frequencies, i.e. high-pitched sounds, as more unpleasant than low-pitched ones. Deep voices, for example, are perceived as sovereign and trustworthy (Eckert 2018).

Younger stands attenuate sound better than old trees. In older stands, the filtering of noise decreases and becomes less and less with increasing tree age. The greatest sound absorption is found in forests with low-hanging branches. A closed forest mantle can increase the sound absorption by another 1–2 dB (A). A stronger effect than same-aged, tall trees is achieved by graded free-grown stands. A noticeable noise-reducing effect is only achieved by forests or forest strips that are 20–40 m, or better over 50 m wide (Flemming 1990). The forest floor is also important for sound absorption. The more irregular the surface structure of the forest floor, the greater the sound absorption.

Road noise, the emission of a line source, is attenuated in the forest to a lesser extent than the noise of a single point source (Mayer 1986). Therefore, it is extremely unfavourable when forests, especially those with older trees, are crossed by roads. Then, noise levels above 50–60 dB, already perceived as unpleasant, are still perceived at 60–100 m from the road in old-growth conifer stands and up to 140 m in old-growth deciduous stands (including pine and larch). Therefore, roads should be at least 400 m away from forest areas that are to remain completely unaffected by road noise (Mayer 1986).

Due to their location and extent, forests have a so-called placeholder effect, by their mere existence, they prevent noise emitters such as roads or industrial plants from being in their area. But noise sources are also present in forests due to management with forestry work. However, only a small area is gerenally affected. Moreover, this noise pollution usually takes place only for a limited period.

Noise is not only a nuisance, it also makes people ill (see Sect. 3.4). Noise protection in forests therefore also plays an enormously important role in keeping people healthy, so that they can rest and recuperate.

Twilight and Forest Colours

The natural illuminance levels in our environment depend on the position of the sun and the conditions in the atmosphere (clouds, dust, haze) as well as other environmental conditions. They vary enormously. The forest also changes the daylight by reducing the diffuse sky radiation and shielding the direct sun radiation when the sun is shining. It is shaded. Illuminance is strongly reduced as a result of the shielding effect of the canopy. On a nice summer day, for example, the illuminance may reach 10,000 lux or more at midday in the open, while in the dense forest it is only 2000 lux. In a normal stand, the brightness is reduced by about 30% on average (Trenkle 1989). A coniferous forest is generally darker than a deciduous forest. In the sparser forest, "light plays" occur, an alternation of light and shade zones.

In addition to the intensity, the spectrum of light is also changed in the forest. The plants and trees absorb the colours of the light in the red and blue range and use them for photosynthesis (Matyssek et al. 2010). Therefore, the green colour is most pronounced and dominates in the upper half-space of the forest. In contrast, the colourful autumn forest results from the withdrawal of water and nutrients from the leaves. However, this varies from tree to tree and leaf to leaf, which is reflected in the variegated autumn colours of the leaves.

In the dense forest, the low light intensity can have a cozy and protective, sometimes also oppressive effect. The differences in colour and brightness, such as a dark green forest in contrast to the surrounding countryside or a colourful autumn forest, have a psychologically stimulating effect (see Sect. 3.4).

Forest Air

The forest air smells pleasantly spicy to humans. The smell comes from the volatile organic compounds that naturally escape in large quantities directly from the plants or the forest floor into the atmosphere (see above). Terpenes or terpenoids form the main component as important essential oils that are responsible for many plant scents (Max Planck Gesellschaft 2012). Coniferous forests are particularly rich in essential oil scents.

For some time now, researchers have suspected that plants "talk" to their neighbours with the help of volatile substances. Recent research has now shown that plants are probably able to transmit, perceive and also understand information about the air or soil to initiate a change in behaviour (Pflanzenforschung 2011). It is also known that plants communicate with each other through various scents such as terpenes or tannins, in which they emit a kind of distress cocktail to ward off enemies. They use scents to attract insects, which then eat an attacking beetle, for example. In the case of parasite infestations, elms and pines also use scents to attract wasps that lay eggs in the leaf parasites in order to use it as an incubator for their offspring (Pflanzenforschung 2011).

But vaporizing an essential oil does not replace a visit to the forest. In a Japanese study (Cheng et al. 2009) it was shown that fresh cedar needles have a considerably more intense terpene content than a distillate made from them. Also, the proportions in the essential oil of cedar needles are significantly lower than in the fresh ones.

Terpenes are inhaled through the respiratory tract during a stay in the forest. Whether they can be beneficial to human health or, perhaps detrimental, is a matter of debate but has not yet been scientifically verified (see Sect. 3.4) and can only be described as speculative at this stage.

Forest Sounds

In the forests, there is generally silence or natural stillness. Nevertheless, special sounds such as the rustling of the forest and the creaking of the trees can be heard, depending on the strength of the wind, in a lighter or stronger form, the cracking of the undergrowth, the babbling of a brook or animal sounds such as the chirping of birds. This shows a positive emotional effect on people (see Sect. 3.4).

Every landscape has its natural sounds (Hedfors 2003), and so does the forest. These are very specific but are also influenced by external conditions. The sounds in the forest, including its sound attenuation, are thus influenced by the season, the time of day and the region in which the forest is located. But weather conditions and other environmental conditions—caused by people in the surrounding area—also play a role (noise from a motorway or industrial plant further away, etc.).

Among the weather influences, wind plays a major role. Although the forest has a protective function against wind, wind sound penetrates the forest to a greater or lesser extent. Weak forest sound is perceived as pleasant, strong whistling or humming, can—together with the visual impression of strong tree movements (sometimes justified, see Sect. 6.1)—make people tense or anxious (Flemming 1990).

Soft Forest Floor

The forest floor is characterised by a soft and elastic texture and is, therefore, more gentle on the joints than urban road surfaces. The elasticity is modulated by different factors such as the moisture of the soil, the type of trees and their root system, and the undergrowth with mosses and plants.

The forest floor (and forest air) also contain an extensive microbiome.

3.2   Sensory Perceptions in the Forest

All our knowledge is based on perception. The five senses are the stewards of the soul.
(Leonardo da Vinci)

Through different relaxation methods, the sensory organs can be addressed and activated anew in the forest. The manifold natural stimuli such as wind sounds or bird calls are predestined to use forest therapy to increase self-awareness.

The human sensory organs are highly specialised organs with which the human being perceives the environment in a differentiated way, evaluates it and can react to it accordingly. In today's predominantly indoor-oriented life, the senses are often not addressed enough and thus reduce or lose their sensitivity. Thus, sensory experiences of nature among children and adolescents, as well as adults, have declined significantly over the past 20 years (Louv 2011). Therefore, it is important and also emotionally enriching to keep the sensory perceptions active, to "train" them or to revive them through external stimuli. A stay in the forest offers excellent opportunities for this.

With eyes, ears, nose, skin and mouth, humans make contact with the environment and receive millions of sensory impressions day after day. The five senses are generally understood to be hearing, sight, touch, smell and taste. Physiologically, these are the visual sense (vision), the auditory sense (hearing including balance), chemical senses such as smell and taste, and the somatovisceral sensory system (including touch) (Lang and Lang 2007).

The human body is equipped with a wide variety of sensory receptors such as thermo, mechano and chemo receptors. The impulses received by these receptors are converted into bioelectrical impulses and transmitted via the nerve pathways to the brain for further processing—only then does the overall impression of the sensory stimulus arise. Certain sensory organs are more strongly linked to the emotional centre in the brain (see below) than others.

The eye is considered to be the dominant sensory organ in humans: this means that the *visual sense* is the most important one. The human eye processes approximately 80% of all information in the environment (Corporate Senses 2018). Using photoreceptors in the retina of the eye, specialised ganglion cells (rods and cones) can perceive different colors, shapes and movements. For depth perception, the left and right eyes each image image differently on the retina. The cells convert the light into energy potentials and transmit it to the brain as optical information. In a special area of the brain (visual cortex) it is processed into a three-dimensional image. Only then is it possible, for example, to estimate distances. Visual stimuli in the form of images are processed very quickly and are subject to weak cognitive control. They can therefore represent strong key emotional stimuli and be used specifically to control attention (Corporate Senses 2018).

A visit to the forest conveys countless visual stimuli that largely harmonise with those from landscape aesthetics (see Sect. 3.3): different tree species, low or high plants and bushes, brown soil with or without vegetation, coarse or smooth tree bark, different shades of green in the changing seasons and the colourful autumn leaves. In winter, snow and ice bathe the forest in cotton wool and leave bizarre shapes and structures on the branches or needles—the forest looks very special, sometimes even mystical. In the sunshine, the light refracted by the trees, leaves and needles forms light and dark, and you see particularly soft colours and plays of light.

However, the sensory perception of "seeing" colours and shapes probably only influences mood and emotions, effects on physical parameters have not been found so far.

In contrast, brightness, i.e. bright daylight, is extremely important for humans. Here, only the light intensity is decisive, because it controls the so-called internal clock. For this purpose, the intensity of the daylight entering the eyes is detected by additional special light receptors in the retina. The information about the light intensity is transmitted from there via nerve tracts to the suprachiasmatic nucleus (SCN). It is located centrally in the hypothalamus and controls the release or inhibition of the hormone melatonin via information to the pineal gland of the brain. Bright light during the day completely suppresses its production. The limit to the biological effects of light is 2000–2500 lux (roughly equivalent to the light intensity on a cloudy day outdoors). The production of melatonin is thus exclusively determined by the incidence of light in the eye and runs inversely, i.e., the darker it is, the more melatonin is produced. This is why melatonin is mainly secreted at night and controls human sleep—which also explains why subdued light intensities or darkness are necessary for sleeping. With lower light intensities, however, melatonin is also secreted during the day and one becomes tired. Even if it is not bright in the morning and during the day in winter or if one remains in a darkened room and bright daylight is missing, melatonin continues to be produced. The person then remains tired during the day, and it may even lead to mental upsets or depressive symptoms (including the so-called winter depression). The internal clock also gets confused, which leads to sleep disorders and other mental and physical complaints (Zulley 2005).

Therefore, for good sleep at night, it is important to be exposed to bright daylight during the day. Conversely, in the forest, the subdued light intensity sets in motion balancing and relaxing reactions.

The second most important sensory perception is *hearing*. Hearing perceives sound waves of different frequencies, which are transmitted to the brain for processing. The sound waves can be received from the environment, but also from inside the body. For example, while eating a crunchy salad, the chewing sounds are picked up and evaluated by the inner ear. In addition to sound frequency and volume, the direction is also analyzed by the brain.

Acoustic stimuli can often trigger strong emotional reactions: A piece of music can move you to tears, a shrill high-pitched voice can be perceived as almost painful, while a gentle soft voice can be perceived as soothing. Sudden noise makes you startle and cover your ears. Noise leads to a reduction in quality of life and chronic illness (Vlek 2005). Sounds can be perceived consciously or unconsciously and can influence well-being positively or negatively.

However, when the sense of hearing is switched off by earplugs (Wooller et al. 2018), mood deterioration occurs. This also happens to a lesser extent when the sense of sight and smell are switched off (e.g. by blindfolds or a nose clip).

Near the sense of hearing is the sense of balance, which analyses the position of the head in space.

Forests, especially the sound-soft forest floor, dampen the propagation of sound (Ziemann et al. 2016). The reduction of noise pollution and the natural quietness of the forest as well as the different natural sounds, create a microclimate that is extremely pleasant for the auditory sense (Hartig et al. 2014). But sounds of "artificial origin", such as from a road running near the forest, make the forest seem less restful (Jahncke et al. 2015), as the auditory stimulus cannot simply be faded out. However, this also depends on an individual's perception of noise. City dwellers affected by daily noise pollution— even though traffic noise can be heard in the background—perceive the same forest as quieter and more relaxing than people living in quiet surroundings. Disturbing noises can be masked by natural sounds (birdsong, rustling trees) and thus be perceived less. This is particularly true for a longer stay in nature, where, during forest bathing, disturbing sounds are increasingly filtered out, as attention focuses more and more on the sounds of nature (Cerwén et al. 2016).

However, these sounds may be only perceived as more pleasant in the forest than in the open, since the perception of (even louder) sounds depends not only on the volume but also on the situation and the mental state (Alvarsson et al. 2010). This is known from music. Bird calls are assessed as restorative in different ways in different individuals. On the one hand, this depends on the type of bird song, and on the other hand, it also depends on the person (Ratcliff et al. 2013).

The *sense of smell* is the most sensitive and complex sense in humans. Unlike the other sensory organs, it cannot be switched off voluntarily (KErn 2015; Hatt 2009), as the nose is part of the respiratory tract and is active for 24 h. It is genetically determined, is also modified by education and experience, i.e. by memories, and is subject to cultural differences.

About 300 olfactory receptors in the nasal mucosa can differentiate around 10,000 different types of odorants (Lang and Lang 2007). The aromas are perceived in two different ways. Either directly via the nasal opening or via the pharynx during chewing. This is why, for example, during a wine tasting, the wine is drawn into the mouth with a slightly open mouth, to address the sense of smell via both perception paths, i.e. more intensively.

The sense of smell is linked to an evolutionarily old part of the brain (KErn 2015) and already warned prehistoric humans of potentially dangerous situations such as smoke or spoiled food. Therefore, odours are very quickly judged by the brain as to whether they represent a danger or not (Pritzel et al. 2003).

However, the olfactory receptors also check a potential partner for suitability or other people in general. The completely correct saying "I can't smell him" is based on the close communication between the sense of smell and the emotional unit in the brain responsible, the limbic system, which evaluates between sympathy and antipathy.

The sense of smell is directly connected to the emotion centre in the brain, therefore perceived odours trigger emotions and memories. This emotional coupling with the sense of smell is described as the Proust effect (Stangl 2018). This effect describes the phenomenon that the human sense of smell can, for example, evoke memories from the long-forgotten past with just a single scent, making it seem as vivid as if it had happened only recently. The typical smell of a forest can thus remind adults in a matter of seconds of childhood visits to the forest.

Apparently, not only the sense of smell and taste but also other organs are equipped with scent receptors (Ravindran 2016). Scent receptors have been detected in the intestinal epithelium, in heart cells, or the bronchial mucus wall, but cancer cells of the intestine or breast also react to different scents (ibid.). This may result in new therapeutic approaches, which are currently being intensively researched (Ruhr Universität Bochum 2018) and could also play a role in forest bathing or forest therapy.

Even in ancient medicine, certain scents were supposed to protect against illness (e.g. the scent of garlic against the plague). Today, in the still-young field of aromatherapy, it is assumed that, for example, lavender exudes a calming scent, the scent of mountain pine stimulates the circulation, lemon scent refreshes and the scent of eucalyptus and thyme is beneficial for respiratory diseases or juniper scent for muscle tension.

Closely related to the sense of smell is the *sense of taste*, whereby about 80% of the perceived taste is actually perceived via the sense of smell. Only 20% is detected by the sense of taste.

A large number of taste buds with sensory cells in the tongue perceive the different tastes such as bitter, sweet, salty, sour and umami (= spicy, savoury) in a differentiated manner (KErn 2015). Further tastes such as fatty, watery or metallic are currently being investigated.

All taste qualities can be felt on the entire tongue as well as in the mucous membrane of the mouth and throat (ibid.). The overall oral impression that is created when a foodstuff is consumed is composed of the taste via the taste receptors of the tongue and the olfactory impression of the olfactory receptors of the nose (= aroma) as well as the physical tactile sensation in the oral cavity (Fillbrandt 2006). In the English-speaking world, the term "flavour" is therefore also used in addition to taste, which encompasses the overall oral impression.

Under particularly favourable conditions at higher temperatures in summer, the forest aroma can also be sensed, together with the sense of smell, via the gustatory taste buds of the tongue.

The somatovisceral sensibility, also known as skin sensation, is perceived by three types of sensory receptors (Lang and Lang 2007). Depending on the location of the receptors in the skin, surface sensitivity, depth sensitivity and viscerosensitivity are distinguished.

The *sense of touch* (surface sensitivity) picks up the quality of touch, pressure and vibration of the skin measured by different mechanoreceptors. The receptor density of the sense of touch is densest at the fingertips, followed by the lips, cheeks and palms/toes.

When touching wood, leaves or a tree bark (see mindfulness exercises in Sect. 5.4.1) or walking on varied soft forest floors during forest bathing, the sense of touch is stimulated to varying degrees—especially when walking barefoot. The sensory impulses from the sole of the foot are transmitted to the brain, where they stimulate the formation of new synapses. This sensory stimulation leads to an increase in brain plasticity, which can improve fine motor skills and harmonise movement patterns (Gisler-Hofmann 2008). A walk over a soft, uneven forest floor can train the sense of balance in addition to the sense of touch, as the forest floor is a perfect refuge for sensory coordination exercises. These exercises are also particularly intensive if you walk barefoot or mindfully or "blindly" for a short distance.

Another skin sensory system is the sense of temperature, which acts via the cold and heat receptors in the skin. The cold receptors are significantly less. The heat receptors in the skin identify local heat stimuli there. More important, however, are those heat receptors located in the brain where they measure the temperature of the blood. This sets in motion actions against overheating of the body (see thermoregulation in Sect. 3.4). The cold receptors are not evenly distributed in the skin, but the highest density is found in the face, here especially in the mouth-nose-throat triangle, followed by the abdomen, and decreases towards the extremities, except fingertips and toes. In addition, surface sensitivity is influenced by a large number of pain receptors.

The *depth sensibility* registers the tension of muscles as well as the stretching of joint capsules and thus enables the sensory quality of proprioception, i.e. the perception of which position the body is in. The soft forest floor provides a good training possibility. If one does additional Tai Chi exercises during the forest bath, the stability is strengthened by the taking place proprioception. Numerous studies with senior citizens (see Sect. 5.4.1) confirm this.

A sense that is negligible for forest medicine is *visceral sensitivity*, which informs about the dilation of hollow organs and vessels as well as about osmotic conditions in order to regulate vegetative functions within the body.

3.3 Aesthetics of the Forest: Why the Forest Is Beautiful?

How beautiful is the forest? Many studies address this question. The basis are studies that generally deal with the visual landscape preference and the resulting recreational effect. The fascination with nature ("wow effect") is the focus of interest. The forest experience and the extent to which the forest appeals to a person, gives him something and he enjoys his visit to the forest, is circumscribed by the term forest aesthetics.

The aesthetic perception of a beautiful forest is fundamentally shaped by the cultural values of a society. However, these are subject to change over time.

The perceptions that a forest is beautiful are subjective and, despite the same cultural background, individually very different and have been shaped by childhood. Nevertheless, for a large part of the population, certain elements make a forest appear "particularly beautiful and appealing".

50 years ago, the German forest was supposed to be "tidy" and well-kept. Today, the aspect of "wilderness" is increasingly coming to the fore (Brämer 2010)—in recent surveys, Germans describe a forest that is as untouched as possible as particularly beautiful (Lupp et al. 2016). However, this is an ideal conception, as there are at most 1% designated wilderness areas in Germany, with a target of 2% by 2020 (Bundesministerium für Ernährung und Landwirtschaft 2017). These are located in the protected areas of nature parks, in parts of the National Natural Heritage as well as in other nature conservation areas. However, 95% of the forests in Germany are cultivated forests close to nature, which at least come somewhat close to this idea of untouched wild nature (Bundesministerium für Ernährung und Landwirtschaft e 2017).

Green nature and forests seem to meet people's colour preferences (although only a few studies have investigated this so far) in terms of mood and emotions (Akers et al. 2012): Even looking at natural forest images has a mood-lifting effect. However, if the forest images are coloured red, they cause rising feelings of anger. Silence and the typical smell of the forest are also part of a beautiful forest.

Likewise, the structures of forests appeal to people: A forest consists of five different levels and is three-dimensional. Branches and twigs create another vertical and horizontal structure. The two lowest levels of the forest is the ground with a layer of soil, covered with a layer of moss and small plants like herbs; the next level consists of shrubs, bushes and young trees, then follows the trunk layer with the branching branches and finally the crown layer. The three-dimensionality and the different levels of the forest form geometric patterns, which are also called fractals or are fractal-like. These are recurring, self-similar patterns that are present in a complex form in all-natural environments but can also be found in architecture or art. These fractal landscapes, which include forests, have a positive effect on people when viewed, leading to an alert but relaxed state (Taylor et al. 2011).

A recent survey investigated forest aesthetics factors in six different regions of Europe. It showed that the desired forest always consists of large old trees with a closed canopy, species richness and different tree species, as well as a low proportion of deadwood and a diverse undergrowth (Ciesielski and Stereńczak 2018).

The *key aesthetic elements* for a beautiful forest describe a mixed forest of conifers and deciduous trees with trees of different heights of different ages and old trees, also solitaires. This forest consists of several species of trees and plants with a great variety of colours. It is crossed by streams, or there are small lakes in it. Different shapes of leaves, plants and trees as well as light treetops, which allow light plays, contribute to the perception of the forest as beautiful. Different structures that create width and narrowness or brightness and darkness appeal to the aesthetic feeling. The ideal forest should also provide beautiful views and vistas into the distance, often opening up new perspectives. Narrow forest paths meander through the aesthetically beautiful forest, leading over soft forest floor. After all, a beautiful forest is also a "clean", waste-free forest.

All the key elements mentioned above, taken together, represent the unique extensive complexity of forest aesthetics and evoke the subjective perception of the beautiful forest. Consequently, the forest per se as a natural space is a potent aesthetic stimulus (Grinde and Grindal Patil 2009). In Germany, this perfectly staged aesthetic natural space is reflected in many forests. In addition to the national parks, forests away from industry and cities are particularly suitable, for example, forests in the German low mountain ranges, the large forest areas on the Mecklenburg lake plateau, the Grunewald, the Havelland, the coastal forests of the Baltic Sea and the forests in the subalpine highlands.

But there are also aspects that some people dislike. These include diseased-looking trees and the amount of deadwood in the forest. It is known that this is an important habitat for animals, but it often disturbs aesthetic sensibilities. Deadwood, like dead trees, gives clues to the ephemeral. Some people do not want to see this, but others find this hint of the finiteness of life enriching.

Over-dense outer forest edges become massive boundaries and are therefore rejected. The aesthetic perception is strongly affected by monotonous forest areas such as spruce stands of the same tree age without gradations in size. They are considered unsightly, as are thickets and shrubby undergrowth that lead to a lack of visibility in the forest. Visible signs of forestry operations, e.g. large logging machines, wide logging lanes, open views of unsightly cut areas, and many downed stumps detract from the image of a beautiful forest, as do chain-link fences, quarries, debris piles, tarred roads, and wind turbines, or off-kind angular building structures within the forest (no log cabin). Wide, straight paths and boundaries are also equally unappreciated.

Noisy forest visitors, mountain bikers and large numbers of visitors, rubbish and human or animal waste in the forest not only impair but destroy the aesthetic perception that the forest is beautiful.

The effect of forest aesthetics on humans depends not only on key aesthetic elements but also on a so-called genetically fixed landscape preference

(Bourassa 1990). Personal positive or negative experiences in the forest during childhood additionally shape one's love or dislike of the forest.

The forest can also gain attractiveness in the course of different life stages (e.g. in childhood), but also lose (adolescence). Thus, for example, a monotonous spruce monoculture can be perceived as a formerly familiar forest as beautiful again.

Even if the key aesthetic elements are present, situational influences play a role (Lupp et al. 2016). For example, the current weather, the season, the type of viewing or even one's own basic mood and feelings modify the evaluation of a forest. The same forest is also perceived differently when it is visited alone or in company.

Thus, the beauty of a forest is judged based on the basic aesthetic key elements, but also always through personal selective perception.

3.4 Health Effects of the Forest Atmosphere

The mechanisms of the health effects of the atmosphere of the forest, which includes not only the forest climate but also the structure and aesthetics of the forest and that we perceive with our five senses, have by no means all been researched.

Excluded from this are the climatic factors of the forest that are relevant to human health. They have already been investigated and scientifically proven, especially in the context of climatotherapy or environmental medicine. In addition, there are at least clear indications for the factors that also belong to the forest climate in a broader sense, that they could also have a positive effect on health. This concerns the light, the colours, the pleasant acoustic stimuli and the haptic experiences. Likewise, the sounds of nature stimulate sensory perceptions and lead to emotional and relaxing effects. The most important effects of the forest atmosphere are:

- Relief from thermal stress: Protection of the thermoregulatory system and the cardiovascular system
- Relief of the airways
- Strengthening through light physical activity and cool air
- Relaxation, calming, well-being

It is unclear whether volatile plant fragrances such as terpenes have a positive effect on health.

The health effects of the climatic factors in the forest are primarily based on the fact that the forest climate is gentle—in contrast to the stimulating climate at the sea or in the high mountains (Schuh 2004). In the case of stimulating climate conditions, the aim is to adapt the body to the strongly pronounced stimulus-intensive biometeorological factors. In a mild climate, the aim is to relieve the body of stressful meteorological conditions or climatic and environmental factors such as air pollution.

Therefore, the forest climate is suitable for general health promotion and prevention. Especially concerning the overstraining demands of our time, the climatic conditions in the forests have a balancing, calming and stress-reducing effect. In addition, the climatic factors of the forests are also effective for many functional disorders and diseases. People who have been exposed to physical or mental stress over a long period of time can be rehabilitated in the gentle forest climate. In general, patients who cannot tolerate any additional strong climatic stimuli are particularly suitable for the forest climate. It offers ideal conditions especially for seniors or very old people, whose regulatory abilities like the performance capacity of thermoregulation are clearly limited. A forest climate is also suitable for very young children as well as for convalescence treatments after serious illnesses and operations who would be overwhelmed by the strong bioclimatic stimuli of the sea or mountain climate. Due to its gentle factors, the forest climate is also particularly suitable for cardiovascular diseases and patients with severe chronic diseases such as airway or malignant diseases.

Relief from Thermal Stress: Protection of the Thermoregulatory System and the Cardiovascular System

Forests offer protection from heat stress and cold, as well as from wind and precipitation (see Sect. 3.1). Compared with a stay in the open land, the demands made on the organism, especially on human thermoregulation, are much lower in the forest.

Humans are so-called homoiothermic creatures. This means that they can maintain their core body temperature, i.e. the temperature of the internal organs and the brain, at a constant 37 °C, apart from minor daily fluctuations. This is possible under changing environmental conditions and with varying own metabolic performance. Maintaining the temperature regulation of the body requires a balance between the heat produced in the body by burning food, among other things, and the heat released into the environment.

The control of the core body temperature and the balance between cooling and overheating is the task of *heat regulation in humans* (thermoregulation). In this process, external and internal signals are collected in the thermoregulation centre in the brain and thermoregulation is primarily activated by variable blood flow to the skin and, if necessary, cold tremors of the muscles or sweat production (Schuh 2004):

In *cold environments,* nerve impulses emitted by the skin's cold receptors cause the skin's blood vessels to constrict (vasoconstriction). This reduces the flow of blood and thus the flow of heat to the surface of the skin. This keeps the heat inside the body and the body cools down only slowly. In the case of severe cooling, muscle tremor sets in for additional internal heat production. This vasoconstriction leads to an increase of blood volume in the core which raises the blood pressure temporarily.

In a *warm environment,* on the other hand, the skin vessels are dilated (vasodilation) and the blood flows through the skin increases. Thus, the heat formed inside the body reaches the skin with the blood flow and is released from there to the environment through various mechanisms. The most important is the evaporation of sweat from the skin surface. In this process, evaporative heat is extracted from the skin, cooling it down. This also cools the blood flowing in the skin so that it flows back into the body core at a lower temperature. This prevents the body core (internal organs and brain) from overheating. If the evaporation of sweat is hindered by clothing or high humidity, for example, the body is no longer cooled sufficiently at high outside temperatures. This then results in a significant strain on the cardiovascular system.

Water evaporation through the skin is a crucial process for heat dissipation and is controlled to a large extent by the humidity of the ambient air.

A measure of the water vapour content of the air is the "relative humidity", which describes the degree of saturation of the air with water vapour. However, the absolute air humidity, the actual water vapour content of the air (vapour pressure), is more important for humans than the relative humidity.

Air temperature and humidity also essentially determine whether a climate or weather situation is perceived as pleasant or unpleasant and stressful (Schuh 2007): High temperatures are accepted as long as the humidity is low. However, if the water vapour content of the air is high, even relatively low temperatures have an unpleasant effect and convey the feeling of *sultriness.* High relative humidity with simultaneous high air temperature hinders the evaporation of moisture from the skin surface, sweat remains on the skin and evaporative cooling is missing. Sultry climatic conditions are thus always a burden on the human body.

Humans perceive the climatic influences on thermoregulation as thermal comfort or discomfort states. The *thermal sensation* of humans depends not only on the measured air temperature, but also on other influencing variables such as wind and air humidity. Precipitation is more likely to be classified as stressful, as it intensifies cold stimuli in a relatively uncontrolled manner, but leads to mugginess and reduced heat dissipation when it is warm. In addition, rainproof clothing often impedes heat dissipation and evaporation, thus possibly leading to an additional burden on heat regulation.

If a person feels thermal discomfort, then he or she tries to regulate it through the behaviour, clothing and posture.

With increasing age, however, humans become more sensitive to heat and cold. At the age of 50, the *tolerance to heat and cold* has already dropped to half, and at the age of 65 only 40% of the youthful capacity remains (Tiedt 1987). This is one reason why, with increasing age, people feel particularly comfortable in the mild forest climate with its balanced temperatures without great heat or severe cold. Also concerning climate change with rising temperatures and more frequent heatwaves, the forest gains even greater importance as a recreational space, because it always remains only slightly warm inside the forest even when outdoor temperatures are perceived as very hot during the day.

But high temeratures in the forest can also lead to sultriness (Höppe and Mayer 1983): due to the higher relative humidity and the reduced wind speed, sweat evaporation can be impeded during physical activity in summer, resulting in thermal stress.

Relief of the Airways

Solid and gaseous pollutants can enter the body and take effect in various ways. However, the main transport routes and contact points are the upper respiratory tract and the lungs. Coarse dust settles largely in the upper airways, throat and trachea during inhalation. It can usually be transported back, i.e. coughed up, by various transport mechanisms. But the smaller particles of the so-called respirable aerosol and the gaseous admixtures such as nitrogen dioxide, carbon dioxide or ozone enter the lungs with the air breathed in and can attack cell structures there.

Air pollutants directly damage and inflame the mucous membranes of the respiratory tract. The frequency of occurrence of respiratory diseases is higher in areas with high air pollution than in non-polluted areas. Numerous studies have found a significant correlation between the frequency of asthma attacks and the concentration of *nitrogen dioxide* (NO_2), as well as for sulphur dioxide (SO_2), hydrogen sulphide (H_2S) and dust particles. Most notably, however, asthma is associated with diesel soot particles, ozone, and tobacco smoke (Behrendt et al. 1997). Other respiratory diseases such as chronic colds and bronchitis are also triggered or worsened by air pollution. It has been known for some time that the effects of individual air pollutants reinforce each other.

Air pollutants also cause an increase in the allergenicity of pollen (Behrendt and Becker 2001).

In addition, the pollutants can pass through the alveoli into the blood and thus cause indirect systemic effects in the body in the form of silent inflammations. They also have an impact on the immune system. It is certain (Fu et al. 2019) that especially the ultrafine fine *dust particles* can lead to an increase in the incidence of cardiovascular diseases, cancer and neurological diseases such as dementia, Parkinson's disease, Alzheimer's disease as well as autism.

Since solid and gaseous air pollutants have a demonstrably harmful effect both on the respiratory tract directly and on the entire body, and can cause numerous illnesses via the so-called systemic effect, the avoidance or relief of air pollutants represents an outstanding preventive strategy. This alone demonstrates the important health-protective effect of the forest.

Strengthening Through Light Physical Activity and Cool Air

In Japanese literature, it is recommended to walk only about 1–2 km during a forest bath of about 2–3 h duration, not to run fast, but to perform Tai Chi, meditation and mindfulness exercises. Whether this can be transferred one-to-one to German mentality, remains to be seen. There are also cultural differences: Walking and hiking are completely unpopular in Japan ("Japanese don't like to hike or walk"). In contrast, many Germans are movement-oriented. *Walking in the woods* is one of them. Physical activity also has an enormous number of health-promoting effects. Therefore, it can only be recommended to move during forest bathing, however not in the sense of a sporty achievement, but the form of relaxed walking or easy hiking. In the spring, autumn and winter months, movement during forest bathing is indispensable anyway, if only to counteract cooling. Gentle walking is also indicated concerning the preventive character of forest bathing.

Above all, the health-promoting physical activity can be carried out in the *cool forest air* with less physical strain than under warm conditions and still lead to a training effect. This is achieved by walking or light hiking in the forest in the form of the well-known and scientifically well-studied climatotherapeutic procedure of climatic terrain treatment (see Sect. 5.4.2). Here, the physical performance and the heat regulation of the person are trained at the same time. The proven effects of the climatic terrain treatment (Schuh 2004) are a significantly increased physical performance, which is indispensable for prevention, and a simultaneous hardening. The advantage is that the effects already occur at low load intensities, i.e. even with relatively slow walking. The climatic terrain treatment fits perfectly with the philosophy of forest bathing and forest therapy, which should not focus on sports in the forest, but on light exercise during relaxed walks and appropriate exercises (see Sect. 5.4.1).

The lower heat load, i.e. the overall cool air inside the forest, can also be used for so-called *training en repos*. This term comes from climatotherapy and can be translated as "training while resting". The fresh-air rest cure (Sect. 5.4.2), which involves lying in fresh, cool air in a quiet place sheltered from the wind, also leads to a slight increase in physical performance, but to a lesser extent than the climatic terrain cure described above. An additional effect is intensive relaxation. This more than 150 years old method is gaining new meaning with forest therapy.

Relaxation and Calming, Well-Being

The *dim light* in the forest interior reduces stress symptoms, also due to a reduction in cortisol levels (Kuo 2015). The subdued light lowers the activity level and allows people to relax. In addition, spending time in a quiet, shady forest covered or "enveloped" by the canopy gives many people a feeling of security. This absence from aggressive environmental and disturbing stimuli and other stressors, including psychological stresses, reduces anxiety. The gentle light and the play of light caused by the refraction of the sun's rays in the canopy influence the mood and can maybe convey a feeling of security.

The dimmed light has not only a relaxing but also a sleep-promoting effect (see below). Depending on the light intensity, the release of the hormone melatonin is controlled, which plays an important role in our psychological well-being. Melatonin affects the mood by calming down and making sleepy, but it can also cause emotional mood swings such as the so-called winter blues. It plays a key role in controlling chronobiological rhythms, especially the day-night rhythm and the seasonal rhythms of humans (see Sect. 3.2).

The twilight in the interior of the forest makes one feel well-tired, calm and relaxed. In addition, it can be assumed that the twilight during a walk in the forest may be helpful to regulate an out-of-sync day-night rhythm (which is often the case in today's world). In addition, physical exercise in the fresh air also makes one tired.

According to the findings of colour psychology, the *green tones* of nature and forests have a relaxing and calming effect. The light conditions prevailing in the forest with the special spectrum have beneficial effects on the psychological sphere (Lichtenfeld et al. 2012) and are very conducive to human well-being.

This is already known from evolutionary research: Nature and forests were elementary for the survival of our ancestors. Green leafy and evergreen forests offered the possibility of protection as well as food resources. This is deeply and unconsciously anchored in humans.

The *smells* in the forest also affect emotional well-being: The typical smell of the forest, which comes mainly from terpenes, damp earth, decaying vegetation and wood, seems to lead to well-being. It is associated by many people with childhood memories and is associated with "nature". It is known from neuropsychoimmunology that positive emotions are directly related to improved immune response. Pleasant smells such as forest air increase IgA formation and reduce cortisol production (Barak 2006). Both parameters indicate a lowered stress level and an improved immune response. The relaxing effect of the forest smell is shown in an experiment: If one smells the essential oil of the two most prominent terpenes (see below), this causes an olfactory stimulation of the parasympathetic nervous system. This relaxation reaction is coupled with a drop in heart rate (Ikei et al. 2016).

Peace and quietness in the forest are more important. Noise is so omnipresent nowadays, and people are not only bothered by industrial or motor vehicle traffic noise but are almost permanently and almost everywhere "sonicated" so that even the term "noise pollution" has been coined (Vlek 2005). Thus, living in an environment in which we are practically permanently surrounded by sounds and a certain level of noise of all kinds, the restorative and regenerative effect of silence is becoming increasingly important. Noise pollution as a daily stressor leads to a reduction in the quality of life as well as to a variety of chronic diseases. Therefore, the EU-wide research strategy of the European network "CALM" calls for the reduction of noise in various areas. The visionary goal of the EU until the year 2020 has been: Avoidance of health-endangering effects of noise pollution on humans and the preservation or protection of quiet zones. Forests—possibly even with designated quiet zones—could thus become an important link in an anti-noise strategy!

Sounds of nature are recommended for relaxation to improve for example sleep disturbances. There is also evidence that patients in hospitals experience a reduction in anxiety, pain and stress when nature sounds are played in their hospital rooms (Cerwén et al. 2016). Various clinical studies showed a calming, anxiety- and stress-reducing effect, and even a reduction in blood pressure was registered when nature sounds were played. Anaesthetised patients react with a stress reduction when nature sounds are played during the procedure (Arai et al. 2008). Nature sounds and the silence typical of forests are perceived as fascinating (Jahncke et al. 2015). This is considered to promote recovery, based on the theory of attention restoration (Kaplan 1987; see Sect. 2.2).

The silence in the woods, animal sounds, single bird calls (e.g. of owls, crows, ravens) or only a slight crackling in the bushes can, however, also be perceived negatively and cause fears, as they are strange, unknown and can create negative associations.

Touching tree trunks or loose wood can also result in a relaxing response. For example, one study showed that when subjects were blindfolded and felt cedar or cypress wood and stroked over it, they experienced a slight drop in blood pressure. Likewise, stroking over a slab of oak wood was shown to result in a relaxing effect (Ikei et al. 2017), the parasympathetic activity increased. In contrast, there was no effect when stroking over marble and artificial materials such as tiles.

The forest is a single large organism consisting of countless living creatures (Suda 2018). The diverse life in the forest (*biodiversity*) that surrounds us when we spend time in the forest also enriches us emotionally. This is supported by the fact that people respond with a stronger relaxation reaction when looking at a living green plant than when looking at a photo of the same plant or an artificial plant (Igarashi et al. 2015).

Possible Health Effects of Phytoncides

According to old Russian studies (Tokin and Kraack 1956), there are hardly any germs in coniferous forests due to the purifying effect of terpenes (for more details on studies, see Sect. 4.3). It is described that the air in coniferous forests had a favourable effect on pulmonary tuberculosis. Therefore, some sanatoria were mostly located in coniferous forests 150 years ago. Whether this can be proven remains to be seen—however, the remarks already show the importance of coniferous forests in healing attempts at that time.

Phytocides (BVOCs such as terpenes, see Sect. 3.1) play a major role in the discussion on the health effects of spending time in forests, especially among the general public. But the state of scientific knowledge on this is still very limited. It is assumed that the effects can be attributed, among other things, to certain plant substances that are found in increased quantities in forests. However, this requires more detailed investigation and replication of studies in non-Asian cultural areas and Central European forests.

Japanese studies show the first indications of the positive effects of phytoncides. For this purpose, several investigations were carried out in the laboratory using a Petri dish: In killer cells, which were weakened by a pesticide, showed a reduced activity, the normal activity could be restored by adding phytoncides into the nutrient solution (Li et al. 2006). Also, natural, unweakened killer cells show a dose-dependent increase in their activity when phytoncides were added to the solution substance. These experiments were additionally carried out in cell cultures as well as in animal models on mice. Finally, in addition to the increase in killer cell activity, a growth inhibitory effect on cancer cells was also observed (Cheng et al. 2009). However, all these effects were dose-dependent, the effect became more pronounced the higher the dose of phytoncides was.

In humans, the impact of phytoncides was considered in a study (Li 2010) in which 12 Japanese people stayed in a hotel in the city for three nights. Phytoncides were vaporised into the air in half of the rooms. An increase in natural killer cell activity and a decrease in adrenaline levels were observed in these six participants after the three nights, but no change was observed in the other six individuals. However, in this pilot study, the concentrations of monoterpenes vaporised into the rooms were many times higher than can be investigated in the forest. Further limiting, an investigation with only 12 participants can at best give the first reference of a possible effect. Therefore, these results must be treated with great caution and can only be taken seriously after confirmation by further studies with larger numbers of test persons and adjusted doses of terpenes.

The significance of phytoncides for health is thus overestimated according to the current state of knowledge. There is a lack of reliable data respective studies to prove sustainable health-promoting effects of terpenes on humans or possible mechanisms of action.

In addition to the discussed but unproven health effects of terpenes and phytoncides, the negative effects of excessive terpene concentrations have been known for some time. Thus, high concentrations of terpenes have been measured in houses with today's modern equipment of natural woods, which apparently can trigger headaches. The cause seems to be the incorrect processing of the wood materials with high solvent concentrations, which can lead, among other things, to mood disorders if there is too little ventilation (Umweltbundesamt 2019).

To date, there are no findings on the health effects of isoprene from deciduous trees.

References

Akers A, Barton J, Cossey R, Gainsford P, Griffin M, Micklewright D (2012) Visual colour perception in green exercise: positive effects on mood and perceived exertion. Environ Sci Technol 46:8861–8666

Alvarsson JJ, Wiens S, Nilsson ME (2010) Stress recovery during exposure to nature sound and environmental noise. Int J Environ Res Public Health 7:1036–1046

Arai YC, Sakakibara S, Ito A, Ohshima K, Sakakibara T, Nishi T, Hibino S, Niwa S, Kuniyoshi K (2008) Intra-operative natural sound decreases salivary amylase activity of patients undergoing inguinal hernia repair under epidural anesthesia. Acta Anaesthesiol Scand 52:987–990

Barak Y (2006) The immune system and happiness. Autoimmun Rev 5:523–527

Baumgartner A (1977/78) Klimatische Funktionen der Wälder. Ber Landwirtsch 55:708–717

Bayerisches Landesamt für Umweltschutz (2015) Luftschadstoffe – Wirkung in Ökosystemen. -https://www.lfu.bayern.de/buerger/doc/uw_39_luftschadstoffe_wirkungen_oekosysteme.pdf. Accessed 20 Feb 2019

Behrendt H, Becker WM (2001) Localization, release and bioavailability of pollen allergens: the influence of environmental factors. Curr Opin Immunol 13:709–715

Behrendt H, Becker WM, Fritzsche C, Sliwa-Tomczok W, Tomczok J, Friedrichs K, Ring JH (1997) Air pollution and allergy: experimental studies on modulation of allergen. Int Arch Allergy Immunol 113:69–74

Beier C, Gundersen P (1989) Atmospheric deposition in a spruce forest edge in Denmark. Environ Pollut 60:257–271

Bourassa SC (1990) A paradigm for landscape aesthetics. Environ Behav 22:787–812

Brämer R (2010) Was ist ein schöner Wald? Naturästhetik als Projektion des Zeitgeistes. https://www.wanderforschung.de/files/schoener-wald1263559879.pdf. Accessed 21 Mar 2019

Bundesministerium für Ernährung und Landwirtschaft BMEL (2017) Waldbericht der Bundesregierung 2017. Langform. Bundesministerium für Ernährung und Landwirtschaft, Bonn

Calfapietra C, Fares S, Manes F, Morani A, Sgrigna G, Loreto F (2013) Role of biogenic volatile organic compounds (BVOC) emitted by urban trees on ozone concentration in cities: a review. Environ Pollut 183:71–80

Cervinka R, Höltge J, Pirgie L, Schwab M, Sudkamp J, Haluza D, Arnberger A, Eder R, Ebenberger M (2014) Zur Gesundheitswirkung von Waldlandschaften. Bericht 147. Bundesforschungs- und Ausbildungszentrum für Wald, Naturgefahren und Landschaft, Wien

Cerwén G, Pedersen E, Pálsdóttir AM (2016) The role of soundscape in nature-based rehabilitation: a patient perspective. Int J Environ Res Public Health 13:1229

Cheng WW, Lin CT, Chu FH, Chang ST, Wang SY (2009) Neuropharmacological activities of phytoncide released from Cryptomeria japonica. J Wood Sci 55:27–31

Ciesielski M, Stereńczak K (2018) What do we expect from forests? The European view of public demands. J Environ Manag 209:139–151

Corporate Senses (2018) Sensorische Reize: Die fünf Basissinne. http://cs.simpel.pl/sensorische-reize/. Accessed 21 Dec 2018

Dietrich HP, Raspe S, Zimmermann L, Wauer A, Köhler D, Schubert A, Stiegler J, Blum U, Kudernatsch T, Klemmt HJ (2018) Umwelt und Standortsbedingungen in raschem Wandel. WLF aktuell 2:6–11

Eckert H (2018) Steht Frauen ihre hohe Stimme im Weg? Interview mit Julia Friese. Welt Wissenschaft am 18(08):2018

Fillbrandt D (2006) Gewürze – die Chemie des guten Geschmacks. In: Experimentalvorträge an der Universität Marburg, Nr. 800. https://chids.online. uni-marburg.de/veranstaltungen/uebungen_ experimentalvortrag.html. Accessed 21 Mar 2019

Flemming G (1990) Klima – Umwelt – Mensch. VEB Gustav Fischer, Jena

Fu P, Guo X, Cheung FMH, Yung KKL (2019) The association between PM2.5 exposure and neurological disorders: a systematic review and meta-analysis. Sci Total Environ 10:1240–1248

Gisler-Hofmann T (2008) Plastizität und Training der sensomotorischen Systeme. Schweizerische Z Sportmed Sporttraumatol 56:137–149

Grinde B, Grindal Patil GG (2009) Biophilia: does visual contact with nature impact on health and well-being? Int J Environ Res Public Health 6:2332–2343

Guenther A (1997) Seasonal and spatial variations in nature volatile organic compound emission. Ecol Appl 7:34–45

Guenther A, Karl T, Harley P, Wiedinmyer C, Palmer PI, Geron C (2006) Estimates of global terrestrial isoprene emissions using MEGAN (model of emissions of gases and aerosols from nature). Atmos Chem Phys 6:3181–3210

Hartig T, Mitchell R, Vries S, Frumkin H (2014) Nature and health. Annu Rev Public Health 35:207–228

Hatt H (2009) Kann man die Nase abschalten? swr.de Blog 1000 Antworten. https:// www.swr.de/wissen/1000-antworten/gesundheit/kann-man-die-nase-abschalten-100.html. Accessed 21 Mar 2019

Hedfors P (2003) Site soundscapes – landscape architecture in the light of sound. Doctor's dissertation, Swedish University of Agricultural Sciences, Uppsala. ISSN 1401-6249

Hehn M, Ziemann A, Ederer HJ, Stüber C, Bernhofer C (2016) Schalldämpfung durch Wald (Teil 2): Vegetationsabhängige Abschirmwirkung von Wäldern – Messtechnische Verifizierung eines akustisch-meteorologischen Modells. Heft 16. Schriftenreihe des Sächsisches Landesamt für Umwelt, Landwirtschaft und Geologie, Dresden

Hewitt CN, Stewart H, Street RA, Scholefield PA (1997) Isoprene and monoterpene – emitting species survey 1997. Biosphere-atmosphere interactions and atmospheric chemistry research group, Department of Environmental Science, Lancaster University. http://www.es.lancs.ac.uk/cnhgroup/download.html. Accessed 20 Mar 2019

Höppe P, Mayer H (1983) Bioklimatische Aspekte des Waldklimas. Z Phys Med Balneol Med Klimatol 12:5–11

Ibrahim MA, Mäenpää M, Hassinen V, Kontunen-Soppela S, Malec L, Rousi M, Pietikäinen L, Tervahauta A, Kärenlampi S, Holopainen JK, Oksanen EJ (2010) Elevation of night-time temperature increases terpenoid emissions from Betula pendula and Populus tremula. J Exp Bot 61:1583–1595

Igarashi M, Aga M, Ikei H, Namekawa T, Miyazaki Y (2015) Physiological and psychological effects on high school students of viewing real and artificial pansies. Int J Environ Res Public Health 12:2521–2531

Ikei H, Song C, Miyazaki Y (2016) Physiological effect of olfactory stimulation by α-pinene on autonomic nervous activity. J Wood Sci 62:568–572

Ikei H, Song C, Miyazaki Y (2017) Physiological effects of touching wood. Int J Environ Res Public Health 14:801

Immich G (2019) Strömungsverlauf des Windes über Wald. Persönliche Abbildung von G Immich, Munich

Jahncke H, Eriksson K, Naula S (2015) The effects of auditive and visual settings on perceived restoration likelihood. Noise Health 17:1–10

Jim CY, Chen WY (2008) Assessing the ecosystem service of air pollutant removal by urban trees in Guangzhou (China). J Environ Manag 88:665–676

Juuti S, Arey J, Atkinson R (1990) Monterpene emission rate measurements from a Monterey pine. J Geophys Res 95:7515–7519

Kaplan S (1987) Aesthetics, affect, and cognition. Environmental preferences from an evolutionary perspective. Environ Behav 19:3–32

KErn – Kompetenzzentrum für Ernährung an der Bayerischen Landesanstalt für Landwirtschaft (2015) Auf die Sinne fertig los. Leitfaden zur Durchführung des Sinnesparcours. Kulmbach. https://www.kern.bayern.de/mam/cms03/wissenstransfer/dateien/leitfaden.pdf. Accessed 21 Mar 2019

Kim JC (2001) Factors controlling natural VOC emissions in a southeastern US pine forest. Atmos Environ 35:3279–3292

Kimmins JP (2003) Forest ecology, 3. Aufl. Benjamin Cummings Publisher, Hawthorne

Kuo M (2015). How might contact with nature promote human health? Promising mechanisms and a possible central pathway. Front Psychol 6:1093.

Lamb B, Gay D, Westberg H (1993) A biogenic hydrocarbon emission inventory for the USA using a simple forest canopy model. Atmos Environ 27:1673–1690

Lang F, Lang P (2007) Basiswissen Physiologie. Springer, Berlin/Heidelberg

Li Q (2010) Effect of forest bathing trips on human immune function. Environ Health Prev Med 15:9–17

Li Q, Nakadai A, Matsushima H, Miyazaki Y, Krensky AM, Kawada T, Morimoto K (2006) Phytonzides (wood essential oil) induce human killer cell activity. Immunopharmacol Immunotoxicol 28:319–333

Lichtenfeld S, Elliot AJ, Maier MA, Pekrun R (2012) Fertile green: green facilitates creative performance. Personal Soc Psychol Bull 38:784–797

Lluisa J, Roahtyn S, Yakir D, Rotenberg E, Seco R, Guenther A, Peñuelas J (2016) Photosynthesis, stomatal conductance and terpene emission response to water availability in dry and mesic Mediterranean forests. Trees 30:749–759

Louv R (2011) Das letzte Kind im Wald. Geben wir unseren Kindern die Natur zurück! Beltz, Weinheim

Lupp G, Rudolf H, Kantelberg V, Koch M, Weber G, Pauleit S (2016) Welcher Wald ist schön? Waldästhetik sucht nach Erklärungen für unser Landschaftsempfinden. LWF aktuell, Nr. 4. https://www.lwf.bayern.de/waldbesitz-forstpolitik/ waldfunktionen-landesplanung/147262/index.php. Accessed 22 Feb 2019

Matyssek R, Fromm J, Rennenberg H (2010) Biologie der Bäume. UTB Uni-Taschenbücher, Bd 8450. Eugen Ulmer, Stuttgart

Max-Planck-Gesellschaft (2012) Ein Katalysator für saubere Regenwaldluft. https:// www.mpg.de/5047427/atmosphaere_selbstreinigungskraft_isopren.   Accessed 20 Mar 2019

Mayer H (1986) Erholungsfunktion von stadtnahen und innerstädtischen Wäl-dern. In: Faust V (ed) Wetter – Klima – menschliche Gesundheit. Hippokrates, Stuttgart

Mayer H (2003) Skript zum Vertiefungsblock „Forstliche Meteorologie" (Block Nr. 222) im Rahmen des reformierten Studienganges Forstwirtschaften an der Universität Freiburg, Freiburg

Meyers Lexikon (1989) Wie funktioniert das? Wetter und Klima. Meyers Lexikonverlag, Mannheim/Wien/Zürich

Mitscherlich G, Schölzke D (1977) Schalldämmung durch den Wald. Allg Forst Jagd-Ztg 148:125–143

Moll WLH (2013) Taschenbuch für Umweltschutz: ökologische Informationen, Bd III. Springer, Heidelberg

Nordrhein-westfälisches Ministerium für Umwelt, Landwirtschaft, Kultur- und Verbraucherschutz. Landeswaldbericht (2019). https://www.umwelt.nrw.de/fil-eadmin/redaktion/Broschueren/   landeswaldbericht_2019.pdf.   Accessed 22 Aug 2021

Nowak DJ, Crane DE (2000) A modeling study of the impact of urban trees on ozone. Atmos Environ 34:1601–1613

Nowak DJ, Hirabayashi S, Bodine A, Greenfield E (2014) Tree and forest effects on air quality and human health in the United States. Environ Pollut 193:119–129

Nowak DJ, Hirabayashi S, Doyle M, McGovern M, Pasher J (2018) Air pollution removal by urban forests in Canada and its effect on air quality and human health. Urb Urb Gr 29:40–48

Pfadenhauer J (1973) Versuch einer vergleichend-ökologischen Analyse der Buchen-Tannen-Wälder der Schweizer Jura (Weissenstein und Chasseral). In: Bugmann H (ed) Waldökologie Vertiefung Wald und Landschaft im Studiengang Umweltwissenschaften. ETH, Zürich

Pflanzenforschung (2011). Wie Pflanzen ihre Nachbarn warnen. https://www.pflan-zenforschung.de/de/pflanzenwissen/journal/wie-pflanzen-ihre-nachbarn-warnen-1540. Accessed 31 Aug 2021

Pritzel M, Brand M, Markowitsch HJ (2003) Olfaktorisches und gustatorisches System. In: Gehirn und Verhalten. Spektrum Akademischer, Heidelberg

Rasmussen RA, Jones CA (1973) Emission of isoprene from leaf discs of Hamamelis. Phytochemistry 12:15–19

Ratcliff E, Gatersleben B, Sowden PT (2013) Bird sounds and their contributions to perceived attention restoration and stress recovery. J Environ Psychol 36:221–228

Ravindran S (2016) What sensory receptors do outside of the sense organs? The scientist. https://www.the-scientist.com/features/what-sensory-receptors-do-outside-of-sense-organs-32942. Accessed 06 Jan 2019

Ruhr Universität Bochum (2018) Duftrezeptor als Angriffsziel für Blasenkrebs-Therapie https://news.rub.de/Presseinformationen/wissenschaft/2018-05-29-riechforschung-duftrezeptor-als-angriffsziel-fuer-blasenkrebs-therapie. Accessed 21 Mar 2019

Schuh A (2004) Klima- und Thalaossotherapie. Hippokrates, Stuttgart

Schuh A (2007) Biowetter. Beck Verlag, München

Sharkey TD, Wiberley AE, Donohue AR (2008) Isoprene emission from plants: why and how. Ann Bot 101:5–18

Smiatek G, Steinbrecher R (2006) Temporal and spatial variation of forest VOC emissions in Germany in the decade 1994–2003. Atmos Environ 40:166–177

Smidt S (1999) Lexikon der forstschädlichen Luftverunreinigungen. FBVA-Bericht 1997; Nr. 199, Aktualisierte Fassung 1999

Smidt S (2004) Waldschädigende Luftverunreinigungen. Eigenschaften – Nachweis – Monitoring – Waldschadensforschung – Immissionsschutz. BFW-Dokumentation Nr. 2. Schriftenreihe des Bundesamtes und Forschungszentrums für Wald, Wien

Stangl W (2018) Proust-Effekt. Lexikon für Psychologie und Pädagogik. https://lexikon.stangl.eu/15875/proust-effekt. Accessed 20 Nov 2018

Steinbrecher R, Hauff K, Rabong R, Steinbrecher J (1997) Isoprenoid emission of oak species typical for the Mediterranean area: source strength and controlling variables. Atmos Environ 31:79–88

Steinbrecher R, Smiatek G, Köble R, Seufert G, Theloke J, Hauff K, Ciccioli P, Vautard R, Curci G (2009) Intra- and inter-annual variability of VOC emissions from natural and semi-natural vegetation in Europe and neighbouring countries. Atmos Environ 43:1380–1391

Suda M (2018) Der Wald ist ein großer Organismus. Persönliche Mitteilung, München. Accessed 06 Dec 2018

Taylor RP, Spehar B, Van Donkelaar P, Hagerhall CM (2011) Perceptual and physiological responses to Jackson Pollock's fractals. Front Hum Neurosci 5:60

Tiedt N (1987) Die Abkühlung – eine physiologische und pathophysiologische Reaktion. Z Physiother 39:255–262

Tokin BP, Kraack E (1956) Phytonzide. Volk und Gesundheit, Berlin

Trenkle H (1989) Wetterfühligkeit vorbeugen und behandeln. Falken, Niederhausen

Umweltbundesamt (2019) Kopfschmerzen. https://www.umweltbundesamt.de/kopfschmerzen-0#textpart-2. Accessed 13 Jan 2019

Vlek C (2005) "Could we all be a little more quiet, please?" A behavioural-science commentary on research for a quieter Europe in 2020. Noise Health 7:59–70

Wagner P, Kuttler W (2012) Biogenes Isopren und sein Einfluss auf die sommerliche Ozonbelastung in urbanen Räumen am Beispiel der Stadt Essen. Posterpräsentation 2012, Fakultät für Biologie, Angewandte Klimatologie und Landschaftsökologie. Universität Düsseldorf, Essen. https://www.uni-due.de/imperia/md/content/geographie/klimatologie/isoprenposter_2012.pdf. Accessed 20 Mar 2019

Wiedinmyer C, Guenther A, Harley P, Hewitt CN, Geron C, Artaxo P, Steinbrecher R, Rasmussen R (2004) Global organic emissions from vegetation. In: Granier C, Artaxo P, Reeves CE (Hrsg) Emissions of atmospheric trace compounds. Kluwer, Dordrecht. www.bai.acd.ucar.edu/Data/BVOC/index.shtml

Wooller JJ, Rogerson M, Barton J, Micklewright D, Gladwell V (2018) Can simulated green exercise improve recovery from acute mental stress? Front Psychol 9:2167

Zemankova K, Brechler J (2010) Emissions of biogenic VOC from forest ecosystems in central Europe: estimation and comparison with anthropogenic emission inventory. Environ Pollut 158:462–469

Ziemann A, Ederer HJ, Stüber C, Hehn M, Bernhofer C (2016) Schalldämpfung durch Wald (Teil 1): vegetationsabhängige Abschirmwirkung von Wäldern – messtechnische Verifizierung eines akustisch-meteorologischen Modells. Heft 16. Schriftenreihe des Sächsisches Landesamt für Umwelt, Landwirtschaft und Geologie, Dresden

Zulley J (2005) Mein Buch vom guten Schlaf. Zabert Sandmann Verlag, Munich

4

Effects of Spending Time in the Forest: Current Studies

Summary

This chapter presents the relevant studies on the short- and long-term health effects of forest bathing and forest therapy. They are scientifically prepared and evaluated. A distinction is made between the relaxing and restorative effects as well as the psychological and physical effects, also on various disease patterns.
If this part seems too scientific, then scroll straight to the conclusion.

In principle, health-promoting and preventive effects are attributed to spending time in nature. Many forest visitors from Asia and from Germany, Austria and Switzerland state in surveys that they go to the forest for health reasons (Roovers et al. 2002). They also describe that stays in the forest are associated with health (Brei et al. 2010), especially due to the clean air and tranquillity (O'Brien et al. 2012), the experience of nature and the distance achieved from daily routine (Hunziker et al. 2012). Likewise, the opportunity to go for a walk or hike is considered important (Zundel and Völksen 2002).

In the individual studies on the benefits of a natural environment available in the international databases, numerous emotional, psychological and physical parameters have been investigated. Most frequently, these are the feeling of recovery, relaxation and well-being as well as the psychological, cognitive and physical effects such as cardiovascular parameters (blood pressure and pulse or heart rate variability as an indicator of regeneration/health). Much less

© Springer-Verlag GmbH Germany, part of Springer Nature 2022
A. Schuh, G. Immich, *Forest Therapy - The Potential of the Forest for Your Health*,
https://doi.org/10.1007/978-3-662-64280-1_4

frequently, the focus is on immunological parameters, physical performance or sleep quality and duration of a forest stay. A few studies have also looked at the effects of Shinrin-Yoku on medical conditions such as ADHD, depression and respiratory diseases.

Research into the health effects of forest visits has its roots in Japan and Korea. For this reason, Japanese studies still dominate the findings on Shinrin-Yoku or forest therapy ("forest medicine"). However, studies from Europe (Finland, Sweden, Denmark, Germany), North America and Australia are now also increasingly dealing with forest therapy.

Almost all studies on forest bathing refer (according to the definition of forest bathing) to prevention. Mostly the stays in the forest were short, some lasted several hours. In a few studies, there was an overnight stay in the forest. Some of them were stays in silence, which is most appreciated by the Japanese, but also stays where a walk was taken in the forest. The results were often compared with those of a control group that stayed in the city in a comparable condition (sitting on a bench, walking in a park, or just strolling in the city) (see Sect. 4.4).

4.1 Recreation and Relaxation

Recreation

In the past, the idea prevailed that recovery is a natural regulatory process that would automatically occur through sufficient break times. More recent concepts see recovery as a bio-psycho-social process through which each individual can take control of his or her mental, physical and emotional health. Allmer (1996) defines recovery as a "stress-regulating and health-promoting resource that enables each individual to deal with stressful situations in a healthy, balancing way and to exert a protective influence on health maintenance". Regeneration through a period of rest after injury or illness is also referred to as recovery. Recovery is thus understood as a reciprocal process consisting of stress (physical, psychological or mental) on the one hand and recovery phases on the other (ibid.). If recovery is lacking, exhaustion, tiredness, sleeplessness and fatigue occur.

Overdemand of the body and psyche/emotions can be caused either by overstraining or also by undertraining. Overload leads to physical and mental fatigue, various stress and tension reactions and finally to illnesses. Constant overload fundamentally disrupts the ability to recover, which shows negative health effects in the long term (Van Hooff et al. 2007). Moreover, studies in occupational psychology show a significantly higher risk of burnout for people with insufficient recovery breaks (Sluiter et al. 1999). Underdemands are often related to monotony or psychological saturation in every day (work) life. Accordingly, depending on the type of stress, different recovery measures are appropriate to recover in the best possible way (Sect. 5.3).

Important factors for nature-based recreation is the enjoyment of nature as well as the letting go of daily stresses (Kaplan 1995). The chance to escape from daily stress, the so-called "being away concept", and perceived privacy are equally important (Cervinka et al. 2014). The recreational effects can be enhanced if the landscape meets individual expectations (see Sect. 3.3).

There is scientific consensus about the recreational and health-promoting effects of decelerating movement activities, body-mind units and active or passive relaxation procedures, which can also be carried out during Shinrin-Yoku.

Relaxation

Relaxation is defined as a "specific physical process that moves along the continuum of activation and deactivation" (Diezemann 2011). A relaxation response leads to a reduction in sympathetic arousal and a modulation of central nervous processes. Physiologically, physical relaxation manifests itself at various levels (Vaitl 2009): There is a decrease in the tone of the skeletal muscles and a reduction in neuromuscular reflex activity. In the cardiovascular system, this leads among others to peripheral vasodilatation, a slight slowing of the heart rate and a reduction in blood pressure. The breathing rate slows down and the breathing cycles become more regular, the oxygen consumption decreases. There are also changes in the immune and gastrointestinal system as well as in the metabolic state.

Regularly applied relaxation procedures promote the individual's ability to relax and thus improve or expand the individual's ability to recover from stressful situations (Fessler 2006). Passive relaxation methods such as sleep, massages or baths have just as much of a recovery-promoting effect as active procedures, although a somewhat stronger effect is attributed to the latter (Allmer 1996).

There are now many different relaxation and body-mind techniques, all of which improve recovery and well-being. People who use relaxation methods to recover regularly in their free time have fewer health problems and psychological exhaustion, less sleep problems and a lower need for rest overall (Sect. 5.4).

Relaxation can take place in different environments: For example in museums, art galleries, monasteries, but also shopping malls and cafés have a proven relaxing effect.

Nature generally offers a particularly pronounced relaxation effect. This was found in a study conducted in England on 4500 people in different regions (Wyles et al. 2017): Stays in nature conservation areas, national parks, rural green surroundings and coastal landscapes lead to a pronounced feeling of relaxation. The improvement in psychological well-being and the associated feeling of relaxation is there stronger than during visits to a city garden or park. Stronger effects were achieved when the visit to nature lasted longer than 30 min.

The mechanism of action of relaxation in nature or forest can be explained via a psycho-evolutionary approach (Ulrich 1979, Chap. 2): In the course of their evolution, humans have developed adaptation processes to different conditions (spatial openness, presence of structures/patterns, water), which together provide the feeling of security and survival.

In a study (Stigsdotter et al. 2017), relaxation during a stay in the forest was compared with a visit to a historic city centre. The forest was additionally equipped with different sensory and perceptual stations that were specifically intended to induce or enhance a relaxation response. In terms of physical parameters, however, no changes were observed in either area. But the feeling of exhaustion and the overall mood in the forest improved significantly. Significant differences were also found between the historic inner city and the forest concerning the perceived recreational effect: The forest was perceived as significantly more relaxing. There was a direct correlation between the decrease in the feeling of exhaustion and the fascinating effect of the landscape. This fits with a second psycho-evolutionary theory, the attention restoration theory (Kaplan and Kaplan 1989), which deals with the fascination of varied landscapes (see Sect. 5.2).

However, even forest-like environments are likely to promote calming and relaxing responses: For example, an improvement in heart rate variability was obtained in elderly Japanese women who spent time on a forest-like planted hospital roof terrace (Matsunaga et al. 2011). Similarly, viewing forest images improved mood and relaxation responses in college students (Song et al. 2018).

4.2   Psychological Effects

Emotional State

Positive mood regulation due to visits to forests and nature is supported by numerous studies. In general, mood regulation is best achieved in a natural environment, as contact with nature increases confidence in oneself (Korpela et al. 2018). A visit to a church in the city was judged to be of equal value.

When "ruminating" about a particular topic, a walk in the woods helps. Brooding is defined as excessive and repetitive thinking about a certain topic. Solutions are rarely found in the process. A walk in nature and the forest (Bratman et al. 2015) reduces this and helps to get off the thought carousel, to think about one's situation in a new and different way and thus find solutions to the problem. Spending time in the forest also improves *mood*: Compared to spending time in the city (Park et al. 2010), a significant reduction in tension, anger, depression and exhaustion can be documented.

A Taiwanese study with elderly subjects investigates the emotion-regulating effects of a 2-h forest bathing programme (Yu et al. 2017). The programme consists of activating four senses (sight, smell, hearing, and touch) while spending time in an alpine forest area. The effects on the mind were consistently significantly positive: Negative moods, anger, hostility, tension and exhaustion reduce, positive mood and vitality increase. Because emotional well-being also operates at the cellular level, an increase in feelings of vitality is associated with stronger immune system defences (Cohen et al. 2006). Finally, forest visits were significantly perceived as anxiety-reducing.

European studies are also increasingly focusing on the effects of forest visits on the state of mind. A Swedish study (Dolling et al. 2017), for example, shows that a twice-weekly visit to the forest for 3–4 h improved the health of stressed individuals in the form of a reduction in exhaustion, stress and burnout symptoms, and better sleep. However, an equally frequent and equally long do-it-yourself-like activity had the same effect as forest bathing. Participants also benefited mentally from both multi-month programmes. They felt more relaxed, more vital and alert, happier, more peaceful and clearer-headed.

Similarly, an improvement in general *well-being* has been documented (Korpela et al. 2018). Since positive impulse control from spending time in nature leads to better general well-being. And the more effectively subjects experience emotion regulation in nature, the healthier they feel. Psychological well-being in natural landscapes, which is closely linked to physical well-being, was measured in England using data from a national longitudinal study of people from over 5000 households 2 years before and 3 years after moving to a city or green space. The results clearly showed that psychological well-being can be influenced by a change of residence. For example, a move to green space caused a spontaneous increase in psychological well-being in the first year, followed by smaller but sustained significant improvements in the three subsequent years. Psychological well-being improved rapidly after the move and remained largely stable over the years. In contrast, when moving to urban areas, there was a decrease in mental well-being initially after the move.

Although there was also an improvement in the three following years, the effects were small and not significant.

Stress Reduction

The complexity and acceleration of life in general, and especially in today's working life, pose special challenges for everyone. Due to technical progress and rapid further development, electronic communication now shapes the everyday lives of most people. Life and work are therefore increasingly under the influence of unlimited, round-the-clock accessibility. In addition to other lifestyle-related influences, this leads to constant stress.

In a recent survey, 11% of Germans state that they are exposed to above-average stress levels, with women being significantly more affected than men (Hapke et al. 2013). It is well known that stress harms numerous body functions in addition to psychological strain and leads to illness. Psychoneuroimmunology has proven that chronic stress, in particular, impairs the immune system. Therefore, a person who is permanently stressed is more likely to become ill.

Nature and the forest reduce stress levels. People with very high chronic stress levels seem to benefit most from forest visits and show a significant reduction in stress (Morita et al. 2007).

Psychological and physiological measurements on Japanese people document that sitting or walking for 15–20 min in forests has a more relaxing effect on the body and mind compared to the same activity in cities. Reduced levels of stress hormones (cortisol/epinephrine) and a switching of the nervous systems to regeneration (Song et al. 2015; Hansen et al. 2017, among others) have been demonstrated. This suggests that even a short stay in the forest can lead to spontaneous stress-reducing reactions. However, it is still unclear whether such a short stay in the forest leads to a sustainable stress reduction that goes beyond the moment.

A Chinese study examined changes in brain activity during a 15-min visit to a bamboo forest compared to brain activity in an urban area (Hassan et al. 2018). 60 subjects were equipped with a mobile EEG device and the results clearly showed that right at the beginning of the forest visit, alpha waves increased significantly and remained at this level. Alpha waves are produced by the human brain when falling asleep, but they can also occur when awake and are described as a state of physical relaxation or rest. When the same participants visited an urban environment the next day, alpha wave activity decreased rapidly. The increase in alpha waves in the forest can thus be understood as a process of mental relaxation, whereas the urban visit is interpreted by the authors as stressful. The significantly stress-reducing effect of a stay in the forest could also be documented analogously based on reduced alpha-amylase values in saliva (e.g. Tsunetsugu et al. 2010).

Numerous studies deal with a general preventive effect of forest bathing due to stress reduction through a stronger emphasis on the parasympathetic activity of the autonomic nervous system. For example, 168 subjects in 14 different forest areas (Park et al. 2011) were compared with city dwellers: A 15–20 min stay in the forest (sitting quietly) or physical activity (hiking in the forest) were studied. Comparable results were obtained in both study designs. Thus, sitting quietly in the forest showed a relevant decrease in cortisol levels, a decrease in sympathicotonic activity and heart rate. At the same time, para-sympathetic nerve activity increased significantly (by 55%). In addition, activity changes were measured in certain brain regions responsible for stress processing (Park et al. 2007). The shift towards more parasympathetic activity, i.e. the calming and relaxing effects of forest bathing, is summarised in a review by Tsunetsugu et al. (2010) with different periods. The relaxation is always shown simultaneously in a reduction of pulse rate and blood pressure values (among others Hassan et al. 2018). Two 90-min forest visits in 1 day showed a reduction in biomarkers of stress (cortisol and immunoglobulin A) (Mao et al. 2012b). In contrast, no change was observed in urban dwellers. Furthermore, stress reduction after 3× 120 min of forest exposure was shown by a decrease in urinary adrenaline levels. This also suggests a parasympathetic response.

These studies are equally confirmed by further studies from the Asian region, but also, from Finland (Karjalainen et al. 2010). Stress-reducing effects of forest therapy were again found in comparison to the urban control group. The relaxing, health-promoting effects were also investigated and proven in South Korea (Shin et al. 2010).

The stress-reducing effects of forest bathing appear to be additionally modified by different personality types (Song et al. 2013). For example, Japanese people with a type A behavioural pattern (winner type, very willing to perform, profit-oriented, aggressive, hostile, stressed, insensitive to the environment) do not react as well physiologically to a forest visit as a person with a type B behavioural pattern (calm, balanced, willing to compromise, stress-resistant). Relaxing, stress-reducing effects such as a reduction in pulse rate were found only in Type B people in this Japanese study. However, forest bathing only took the form of sitting for 15 min. It can be assumed that Type A people just simply need a longer time to relax. This is also described in the psychological literature on the Type A personality.

In their study of almost 500 young, physically healthy Japanese, Morita et al. (2007) documented positive effects on the psyche. After only 2.5 h in the forest, the subjects showed a significant reduction in depressive feelings, hostility, and fear compared to the control group. At the same time, there is an increase in a feeling of "more liveliness". This study also underlines that the forest environment exerts positive effects on the psyche. The mood-lifting effect of spending time in the forest is stronger the greater the mental strain on the individual.

Even in the case of severe stress-related symptoms such as burnout, a stay in the forest can be effective. A study of patients in a stress clinic concluded (Sonntag-Öström et al. 2011) that forest stays and therapeutic interventions in forest landscapes can support the treatment of stress-related exhaustion very well.

However, relaxing, stress-reducing reactions can also be generated in humans virtually: a 3-D film about a forest, with nature scenes from inside the forest and the corresponding sounds, leads to a parasympathetic reaction in the viewers, which has a stress-reducing effect (e.g. Annerstedt et al. 2013).

In summary, the studies show that spending time in the forest dampens the activity of the sympathetic nervous system and particularly stimulates the parasympathetic nervous system. This has a relaxing, stress-reducing effect (Meyer and Bürger-Arndt 2014). Overall, it can therefore be confirmed that spending time in the forest has a stress-reducing and mood-improving effect. A stay of several hours in the forest seems to be sufficient for this effect. According to a recent study, at least 2 h, and preferably up to 5 h/week are effective (White et al. 2019). Thus, for health promotion and general prevention, and especially in terms of stress reduction, it must be recommended that forest visits lasting several hours carried out regularly and repeatedly at short intervals per week!

Cognitive Effects: Memory and Attention Performance

People remember images of natural landscapes better than images of cities (Berman et al. 2008).

Comparing cognitive ability and attention in nature with those in the city, there is a significant improvement in memory and attention performance after a walk in the forest. At the same time, the subjects who took a walk of about 50 min in a forest/park feel refreshed. In contrast, there was no improvement after spending time on busy inner-city streets (ibid.).

Noise and sounds interfere with memory performance, but in a quiet forest, the memory performance increases. If test subjects see pictures or films of natural landscapes, but at the same time hear urban traffic noise or voice confusion during a memory test, then the urban traffic noise impairs the memory task. In contrast, only viewing nature images in combination with the typical sounds in the forest does not lead to any impairments and does not interfere with memory performance (Benfield et al. 2010). Some US national parks are already reacting to this result by trying to minimise subliminal traffic noise and thus enable visitors to enjoy a significantly higher recreational effect.

These findings on memory performance are supported by a large number of studies based on Kaplan's (1995) "attention restoration theory": Pleasant and intriguing stimuli, e.g. a sunset or light reflections in a forest, lead one to be relaxed-attentive. In contrast, sudden stimuli in the city (car horns) induce an immediate stress response.

The elderly enjoy nature most when they can experience it. They are sitting and observing nature, and preferably still in the community (Orr et al. 2016). The seniors enjoy the beauty of nature and draw strength and vitality from it. The multisensory experience of nature plays a major role in this—fresh air, sunshine and colourful natural landscapes are all part of enjoying nature. Dementia patients in particular benefit from spending time in nature and show improved sleep quality and an increased sense of well-being (Orr et al. 2016), and the memory capacity of patients with dementia also increases (Whear et al. 2014).

Even school performance can be favourably influenced by a tree-rich environment (Sivarajah et al. 2018): The closer and denser the trees are to the school, the better the school performance. Thus, a green environment not only makes one healthier but also enhances cognitive performance.

Mental Illnesses

It seems that therapy in nature has beneficial effects for patients with depression. That is why today a forest is often used as a therapy room in the treatment of depressive patients. For example, behavioural therapy conducted in the forest shows better results for depressive patients than the same therapy indoor in a hospital (Kim et al. 2009). A nine-day forest camp for depressed former alcoholics also documented a significant improvement in psychological well-being compared to standard treatment in a randomized controlled trial, and the patients were also sleeping better (Shin et al. 2012). Psychologically more stressed persons achieve a greater improvement.

Specific programmes of forest therapy for depression consist mainly of walking in the forest, supplemented by forest experience with the five senses, Qigong, forest contemplation, forest meditation, aromatherapy, herbal tea therapy and handicrafts with natural materials.

The benefit of such programme is demonstrated by a high-quality meta-analysis of 28 randomised intervention studies (with a control group), which surveyed the effects of different forest therapy programmes in depressive patients (Lee et al. 2017). Although the length and duration of the forest stay and the programme content differed in the individual studies, the result of the analysis shows that depressive patients can generally experience an improvement through forest therapy.

Stroke patients or cardiac patients suffering from depression or anxiety also experience a reduction in symptoms during a four-day forest therapy programme. Forest bathing or forest therapy can therefore definitely be recommended as a complementary or alternative therapy option for these patients (Chun et al. 2017).

4.3   Physical Effects

Overall, only a few studies deal with the treatment of existing diseases in the forest, since forest bathing or forest therapy and forest medicine have so far mainly been oriented towards prevention.

According to current knowledge, a one-time, short-term stay in the forest does not seem to have any lasting physiological effects—apart from the possible acute stress-reducing effects mentioned above. This is indicated by a systematic review (Bowler et al. 2010), which evaluates the benefits or effects of green spaces/parks/forests in comparison to urban environments (with the same activities). It shows that for short durations of less than 1 h (e.g. walking, hiking or jogging) no evident positive physical effects on health or well-being can be proven. Thus, more extensive, higher-quality studies (see Sect. 4.4) are required to demonstrate physical changes resulting from short stays in the forest.

In the case of stays of several hours in the forest, the data situation promises rather physical effects, yet these are large effects in the preventive sense. Concerning individual *preventive physiological effects,* the data situation is as follows:

Blood Pressure
In numerous studies in which young, healthy participants (mostly students) were examined, short-term blood-pressure-lowering effects were described in isolated cases even with a stay of only 15 min (Hassan et al. 2018), but in other studies with several stays in the forest, no blood pressure-regulating effect was documented (Morita et al. 2011a). This is not surprising, as the blood pressure of the young healthy volunteers should have been in the optimal range anyway.

In contrast, older people who walk in the forest for 90 min in the morning and 90 min in the afternoon show a significant reduction in blood pressure (Mao et al. 2012a). A blood pressure-lowering effect can also be documented in middle-aged people (Ohe 2017): Office workers (20–60 years old, two-thirds women) with normal-high blood pressure or borderline elevated blood pressure (above 120 mmHg) were studied. After 1–5 days of staying in the forest and experiencing forest bathing, there was a reduction in blood pressure that lasted for 3–5 days. Individuals with borderline hypertension achieved greater overall improvements than individuals with normal blood pressure. Consequently, people with mild hypertension benefit particularly from the relaxing effect of forest bathing when staying 1,5 days in the forest (Ohe 2017).

A South Korean study came to the same conclusions (Lee and Lee 2014). After a 1-h walk in the woods, the blood pressure of the older female subjects drops significantly compared to the control. At the same time, lung capacity and the elasticity of the arteries improve.

Finally, a current systematic literature review including a meta-analysis summarizes the various studies on forest therapy and blood pressure behaviour. The authors attest that spending time in forests shows a significant positive blood pressure-lowering effect (Ideno et al. 2017). Thus, it can be assumed that the above-described, clearly established stress reduction through forest visits also affects systolic blood pressure.

Spending time in the forest also appears to have the potential to delay the development of atherosclerosis. The first indications of cardio-protective effects are provided by the above-mentioned study (Lee and Lee 2014) with 40 people in each case. In normal-weight female seniors, there is a measurable physiological relaxation response in the vascular system. In contrast, the comparison group in the city experiences a deterioration in all cardiovascular parameters. Chronic and oxidative stress, as in the city, promotes the development of vascular calcification. Forest stays regularly, can also have a health-protective effect concerning the development of atherosclerosis.

For the Japanese, on the other hand, the mere sight of a forest is enough to cause a reduction in pulse rate and blood pressure (Song et al. 2013). It can be assumed that this pronounced reaction is due to the hectic and stressful life in Japanese cities and the different cultural background.

In summary, forest bathing for several hours achieves a reduction in blood pressure, especially in people from middle age with slightly elevated blood pressure values. This is an important preventive factor of forest bathing! Spending time in the forest thus reduces the risk of cardiovascular disease by lowering blood pressure. "Forest bathing" consequently promotes cardiovascular health.

Immune System

There is intensive discussion in the scientific literature and among the general public whether spending time in the forest can lead to favourable changes in the immune system with all the positive consequences for the prevention or healing of a wide range of diseases. If there are effects on the immune system, it can be assumed, according to the current state of research, that the high air quality in the forest as well as the reduced stress level and relaxation in the forest due to physical activity or quiet exercises in the natural environment play the most important roles. There are also indications that an increase in parasympathetic activity alone could lead to an increase in the activity of killer cells. Favourable effects of forest visits on the immune system are found in an increase in immunoglobulins A, G, and M (Ohira et al. 1999) and a decrease in stress hormones in healthy subjects (Li 2017). Thus, forest visits can have a positive effect on the immune system.

However, the phytoncides of conifers can also be considered as active substances on immunological parameters—in Asian literature, a positive effect of terpenes in particular on the immune system is frequently reported. But the state of scientific knowledge on this subject is still very limited or even contradictory (see Sect. 4.4):

The discussion focuses on the studies of the Japanese Professor Li. He examined 13 healthy nurses who spent 3 days and two nights in a forest environment (Li et al. 2008a). Measurements of natural killer cells (NK cells), T cells and stress hormones were taken before the stay, on the second and third day in nature, and seven and 30 days after the return to normal life. In all subjects, there was a significant increase in natural killer cell activity and a significant reduction in the stress hormones adrenaline and noradrenaline. Both improvements could still be measured after 7 days. A follow-up study (Li et al. 2007, 2008b) examined immune reaction in 12 men who spent 2 h in the forest twice a day for 3 days: Natural killer cell activity increased, and concentrations of the stress hormones epinephrine and norepinephrine dropped significantly. The increased level of NK cells could still be detected after a further 7 days. A day trip into the forest yielded the same result (Li et al. 2010). Since the three studies come to the same conclusion, there seems to be no difference in the immune response between repeated 2-h and multiday forest visits. Thus, one could conclude from Li's studies that for a possible stimulation of the immune system in healthy individuals—if at all due to the small number of participants (see Sect. 4.4)—a forest stay of several times and several hours (of at least 4 h each) must take place. However, a Chinese research group (Mao et al. 2012b) repeated Prof. Li's last study and could not confirm his killer cell results. Moreover, COPD patients responded with a significant decrease of intracellular perforin levels (a NK protein) after several days of forest visits (Jia et al. 2016). In contrast, in a Korean forest bathing study in patients with chronic pain syndrome, the forest atmosphere stimulated killer cell activity (Han et al. 2016).

The results on how forest bathing affects the activity of killer cells are thus contradictory. Therefore, in principle, the finding that the activity of natural killer cells in the body is increased by spending time in the forest—and specifically due to the presence of phytoncides—and that this effect even lasts for a few days, must be seriously questioned from a scientific point of view. Claims circulating in the media that exposure to phytoncides during forest visits can even protect against cancer must also be regarded as unscientific and speculative at present (see Sect. 4.4).

However, there are also more recent studies that have the advantage that they were conducted with slightly more subjects (see Sect. 4.4) and survey other immune parameters. For example, a study with 36 patients suffering from chronic cardiac insufficiency demonstrate the positive effects of spending several days in a forest (Mao et al. 2018): Within 1 month, the patients spent 4 days and nights in a Chinese forest once or twice. Inflammatory mediators such as TNF-α, BNP, cytokines and oxidative stress, which are often elevated in patients with chronic heart disease, decreased significantly after the forest stays. In a previous study, Mao et al. (2012a) were already able to indicate the positive effects of a forest stay in cardiac patients, as there had been an improvement in the inflammatory parameters of the vessel walls. In summary, these two studies provided the first evidence of additional health benefits from forest visits in chronic heart patients. Im et al. (2016) also demonstrated the same health-protective results in a controlled study during a 2-h stay in the forest compared to an equally long stay in the city in 40 people in each case: Subjective stress levels and the immune values involved in inflammation were reduced by a visit to the forest.

It is also speculated (Yatsunenko et al. 2012) that the interaction of microbes from the forest air or, in particular, the soil of the forest floor could affect the immune regulation of humans. Background are studies that showed that children, who grew up in a rural environment with appropriate natural pollution, develop fewer allergic diseases than children living in the city in an environment with fewer microbes (von Mutius 2019). Consequently, a more or less sterile environment seems to be conducive to inflammation in different chronic diseases (Hanski et al. 2012, among others). There is also evidence that urban-dwelling people have a lower diversity of gut microbiota than people with a lot of nature contact (Rook 2013). The extensive natural forest microbiome might interact with the skin as well as the respiratory tract. Both are involved in immune regulation along with the gut microbiome (Flandroy et al. 2018). Thus, contact with the forest microbiome could contribute to the natural harmonisation and regulation of the immune system. However, it is important to note that microbes can also make one sick (Chap. 6).

Sleep Quality

The influence of forest visits on sleep quality and sleep disorders was investigated in a Japanese study involving 71 physically healthy subjects with sleep disorders who completed a forest walk for 2 h each over 8 days (Morita et al. 2011b). Significant improvements were achieved in all sleep parameters measured on the nights before and after the walk (sleep duration, depth and quality, and nocturnal movement or restlessness). In addition, a walk in the forest in the afternoon was found to have significantly more positive effects on sleep patterns than in the morning. Persons with sleep disorders thus have a significant benefit if they walk in the forest for 2 h in the afternoon. The reason for this may be stress reduction, but also physical exercise during the forest walk. Another study also shows an increase in sleep duration during the forest bathing programme, although this was only carried out with 12 people (Kawada et al. 2012).

Body Mass Index (BMI)

A Californian working group conducted a multicentre study of people's access to green spaces/parks/forests over 7 years and was able to document a correlation between a reduction in BMI and the number of visits to parks (Stark et al. 2014). The underlying reason is probably that the use of nature, for example, in the form of a nearby forest, promotes physical activity and thus increases the metabolism.

Manifest Diseases

A large number of studies prove clear preventive effects of forest bathing on blood pressure and sleep quality. The impact mechanism seems to be at least indirectly via the stress-regulating and recovery-promoting effect on the immune system.

Recently it has been investigated more frequently whether manifest clinical pictures respond to forest bathing or forest therapy (depression see Sect. 4.2). These include:

Respiratory Tract Diseases

People who are constantly exposed to high levels of air pollutants (see Sect. 3.4) benefit from the relieving conditions in forests. Patients suffering from bronchial asthma, chronic bronchitis or chronic obstructive pulmonary disease (COPD) need clean air to prevent their condition from worsening. However, due to today's environmental conditions, clean air is almost only be found in forests.

In 20 patients with chronic respiratory disease (COPD), a decrease in all inflammatory parameters was found after a forest visit lasting several days, whereas these parameters increased in the urban comparison group (Jia et al. 2016). The authors explain this effect as a strong relief of inflammatory stimuli (air pollutants) through the forest visit, which has a positive effect on the respiratory capacity and in the form of a reduced physiological stress potential after the forest stay.

A four-day forest education stay showed a significant improvement in Korean pupils diagnosed with bronchial asthma or atopic dermatitis (neurodermatitis or psoriasis) (Seo et al. 2015). The clean air in the forest is also a relief for these diseases, because air pollutants promote inflammation in the body and further activate the already hyper-reactive immune system (see Sect. 3.4). This may also manifest itself in a worsening of the skin condition (Vocks et al. 2001).

Patients suffering from the chronic obstructive pulmonary disease who additionally underwent forest therapy five times during a three-week rehabilitation stay at the Baltic Sea showed improvements in several clinical parameters compared to the control group, whose members underwent a comparable indoor programme (Kaiserbäder Insel Usedom 2018).

Cancer

The references to the positive effects of forest visits for cancer patients that appear again and again in the numerous books and articles on forest bathing have so far not been substantiated in any way. They are only based on assumed connections between the effects of forest visits on the immune system (see above) and the development of cancer. To date, there are no valid studies on this subject! Although a pilot study provides initial indications that breast cancer patients who have undergone surgery can experience an immune stimulation through a 14-day forest therapy (Kim et al. 2015), no statements in this direction should be made here based on the current state of knowledge, and thereby possibly raising false hopes (see Sect. 4.4)!

Nevertheless, psychological relaxation, clean air and physical exercise, as well as body-mind or mindfulness exercises, are good for convalescence or aftercare of cancer patients. For each of these listed items, the positive effects are known or proven. Women with breast cancer are said to recover better (Cimprich and Ronis 2003), and their sense of well-being seems to increase when getting in contact with nature (Nilsson et al. 2011). Therefore, a stay in the forest can be recommended as an individual coping strategy.

The extent to which cancer patients use nature as a helper and comforter was investigated by a Swedish research group (Ahmadi and Ahmadi 2015). The results of approximately 2500 Swedish cancer patient surveys showed that nature and forest visits represent an important coping strategy during and after cancer treatment. Sounds of nature such as birds chirping or wind sounds are likewise described as an important coping tool (ibid.). Finally, cancer patients consider natural spaces as an important "nurturing" and familiar refuge (Blaschke 2017). For example, a mighty tree can provide emotional security in times of existential crisis. Thus, a regular visit to the forest can help patients with cancer to better bear the burden of the disease.

Attention Deficit Hyperactivity Disorder (ADHD)
When children with ADHD spend time in green spaces, impulsivity and attention deficits are reduced compared to spending time at home or in urban environments (Kuo and Faber-Taylor 2004). After a 20-min walk in a park, compared to an equally long walk in the city centre or a residential area, the symptoms of hyperactive children suffering from concentration disorders decrease significantly. The strength of the improvement is comparable to the effect of a drug (ibid.).

Thus, nature visits in the form of nature or forest kindergartens, which are popular in Germany, are particularly useful for hyperactive children.

Pain
Initial indications for positive effects of forest stay on pain reduction are provided by two Korean studies: A 5-day forest bathing programme can reduce pain as well as the number of trigger points in chronic neck pain. However, it is particularly effective when the programme consists of a combination of forest bathing and exercise therapy in the form of stretching and strengthening (Kang et al. 2015). General chronic pain syndrome was also improved during a 2-day forest health programme (Han et al. 2016). In addition to 2-h forest bathing, the pain patients were instructed with various programmes such as music therapy, mindfulness exercises, as well as learning sessions on pain management, whereas the control group spent their daily lives unchanged. Not only did the pain decrease, but the psychological state and well-being also improved significantly as a result of the visit to the forest.

Autism

The fact that nature has a positive effect on autistic children has been documented by a study of Californian primary school pupils: Nearby wooded areas, for example, but also green streets seem to exert a certain protective factor against autism (Wu and Jackson 2017).

Indications can be found in a survey of affected parents (Li et al. 2019). According to this, autistic children benefit particularly from an improved sense of movement, but their emotional and social well-being are also improved. However, parents also see clear barriers to going outdoors with their children: Safety concerns, fears and unforeseen behaviour of the children as well as possible reactions of society.

Other Diseases

Finally, a few studies also focus on the therapeutically use of forest stays for several chronic diseases such as cardiac insufficiency, addiction or post-traumatic stress disorders. So far, however, they only provide initial indications of a possible beneficial influence of forest therapy on these clinical pictures.

A review that evaluated different studies with healthy individuals or patients (Oh et al. 2017) during forest stays between 1 day and 11 weeks concludes that forest bathing or forest therapy is largely risk-free and hardly any relevant side effects are to be expected.

Living Longer and Healthier in a Forest Environment?

People who live near forests are said to be healthier and live longer, according to some research.

A pioneering nationwide Danish population study with data from over 900,000 Danes can be used as a basis for this claim: Thereby it was documented how important green spaces are during child development for later healthy mental development (Engemann et al. 2019). Children who had little or no green space in their living environment by the age of 10 showed up to a 55% increased risk of developing a psychiatric disorder in adulthood. In contrast, data shows that the greener space there is, the more health-protective this is for later life. This is also confirmed by other epidemiological studies, which clearly show that a higher proportion of green spaces in urban areas leads to better general well-being and has a positive effect on the health of the population.

About living near a forest, a study from Berlin (Kühn et al. 2017) can demonstrate that living near a forest (and also near a water landscape) is an important factor for health! Children who live and play near large wooded areas have fewer chronic diseases. Their psychological development is also more stable (Kuchma et al. 2008). A large-scale American study of over 5000 subjects in and around Washington City (Akpinar et al. 2016) documented that the more forested areas nearby, the fewer days of sick leave due to mental illness occur. Further evidence that living in, near, or spending frequent time in the forest has a longer-term positive effect on cardiovascular health is provided by a Taiwanese study (Tsao et al. 2014) of forestry workers who had been in their job as foresters for at least 1 year, compared with urban workers in metropolitan Taiwan. Various measured parameters such as blood lipids or blood glucose showed that the foresters had significantly lower cardiovascular risk factors, even though their alcohol consumption was three times higher than that of the urban workers. This may be due to the lifestyle in the forest, but also to the lower pollution by nitrogen oxides and fine dust.

Living or spending a lot of time in a green environment, which of course includes being near a forest, is also thought to reduce mortality, especially from cardiovascular disease—this was found in a study from England (Mitchell and Popham 2008). Similar results were also found in studies from the Netherlands and Finland (Maas et al. 2006), where a daily visit to the forest had the strongest health effects (Sulander et al. 2016). More forested areas close to home mean fewer unexpected deaths (Wu et al. 2018). A Japanese epidemiological study examined the association between forest areas and cancer-related deaths. In addition to gender differences, the authors were able to show a dependence on forest density: If forest areas occupied more than 60% of the living environment, the standardized mortality rate for female breast cancer and prostate cancer decreased (Li et al. 2012). Furthermore, high forest richness leads to fewer deaths from lung and uterine cancer in women and kidney and colon cancer in men.

A study from the United States of America has also established in a calculation model that the reduction of forest areas in the immediate living environment leads to an increase in mortality from cardiovascular and respiratory diseases. The authors (Donovan et al. 2013), however, qualify the statement of this result to the effect that they only want their study to be understood as an indication of the importance of forests for health.

Overall, however, it appears that living in forest environments has health-promoting effects and may even confer a survival advantage.

4.4   Limitations from a Scientific Point of View

The existing studies on Shinrin-Yoku can be divided into two groups: Experimental studies on the stay in forests and laboratory studies investigating individual effect factors of the forest (such as phytoncides). Only in the experimental studies are occasional some studies with sufficiently large numbers of cases and valid statistics available.

In most Japanese studies, a comparison has been made between spending time in the forest and spending time in an urban environment (Japanese cities). However, these are situations that cannot really be compared because the conditions are completely different in terms of air quality, thermal conditions, noise, etc. Even if the control groups were in an urban park or forest area in the city, it can be assumed that this is different from a natural forest in terms of tree population, density and size alone. In addition, studies have often included different groups of people rather than the same ones—for example, urbanites and rural dwellers, who may have completely different perceptions. This is particularly problematic when psychological or emotional parameters are being studied. In the existing studies, the subjects spent the forest stay in groups and not alone. The question must be asked here whether social interaction and the group experience do not also influence psychological well-being. It is therefore not known whether a visit to the forest in small groups or alone is more beneficial.

Finally, the supposedly positive study results on the health effects of forest bathing are also particularly limited by the fact that almost all studies were only able to document a short-term change in the parameters. This was because the parameters studied were usually only measured at the end of the forest stay and only rarely after one or several weeks. Therefore, only a statement about the short-term gain for health is possible. There is hardly any knowledge about whether and how long the effects last after the forest stay has ended.

In the existing studies, forest bathing or forest therapy is mostly combined with physical activities such as walking or hiking. However, physical activity has—and this is clearly proven—the same health-promoting effects that are attributed to spending time in the forest. The short-term effects of physical activity on physical and emotional well-being and the psyche have also long been proven. Therefore, in the final analysis, it is not clear how large the proportion of the forest and its atmosphere is in comparison to the amount of physical activity. One cannot rule out the possibility that the measured effects are caused by activity alone.

Concerning the discussion about the influence of phytoncides (terpenes) on the immune system, it must be assumed that although there are indications of a possible influence, there is still no reliable evidence of real connections. The interpretation that forest bathing should therefore be used to prevent cancer is unjustified based on the current state of knowledge.

Furthermore, there are no clear findings on how often, with what frequency and time intervals forest visits must take place. About the length of a forest stay, it can at least be assumed that a stay of several hours is sufficient to achieve the short-term effects described above.

Finally, the question arises as to which elements or structures in the forest caused the health benefits. Are there individual factors or the interaction of all of them? Furthermore, it is not yet clear how the impact differs in various natural areas. And finally: How must a stay in the forest be designed so that it optimally serves various health purposes?

4.5   Conclusion: Is Forest Therapy Beneficial to Health or Healing?

Forest therapy has proven effects on physical and mental health. It is health-promoting and particularly suitable for general prevention and in cases of stress-related strain. This is confirmed by the studies listed above. The results concerning stress reduction should be emphasised: During stays in the forest for several hours, there is an increase in parasympathetic activity, which plays a very important role in recovery and relaxation. This can be seen in blood pressure and heart rate and other parameters. Beneficial effects on the immune system are also possible. Forest therapy lifts the mood and improves psychological well-being.

Forest therapy reduces the known risk factors for cardiovascular diseases. The quality of sleep is improved by an afternoon visit to the forest. Spending time in the forest can counteract a worsening of respiratory diseases and can be used as an adjunct in the treatment of depression and cancer. However, healing aspects for existing diseases have not been proven.

Larger forest areas, as well as forest therapy, are thus of great and increasing importance for human health and well-being. It can be assumed that isolated visits to nature or the forest will probably only have short-term effects in terms of relaxation, whereas regular visits to the forest or living "in the green" will bring lasting health benefits.

References

Ahmadi F, Ahmadi N (2015) Nature as the most important coping strategy among cancer patients: a Swedish survey. J Relig Health 54:1177–1190

Akpinar A, Barbosa-Leiker C, Brooks KR (2016) Does green space matter? Exploring relationships between greenspace type and health indicators. Urban For Urban Green 20:407–418

Allmer H (1996) Erholung und Gesundheit. Hogrefe, Göttingen

Annerstedt M, Jönsson P, Wallergård M, Johansson G, Karlson B, Grahn P, Hansen ÅM, Währborg P (2013) Inducing physiological stress recovery with sounds of nature in a virtual reality forest – results from a pilot study. Physiol Behav 118:240–250

Benfield JA, Bell PA, Troup LJ, Soderstrom NC (2010) Does anthropogenic noise in national parks impair memory? Environ Behav 42:693–706

Berman MG, Jonides J, Kaplan S (2008) The cognitive benefits of interacting with nature. Psychol Sci 19:1207–1212

Blaschke S (2017) The role of nature in cancer patients' lives: a systematic review and qualitative meta-synthesis. BMC Cancer 17(1):370

Bowler DE, Buyung-Ali LM, Knight TM, Pullin AS (2010) A systematic review of evidence for the added benefits to health of exposure to natural environments. BMC Public Health 10:456

Bratman GN, Hamilton JP, Hahn KS, Daily GC, Gross JJ (2015) Nature exposure reduces rumination and subgenual prefrontal cortex activation. PNAS 112:8567–8572

Brei B, Heiler A, Claßen T, Hornberg C (2010) Gesundheitsressource Stadtgrün – gesundheitswissenschaftliche Implikationen für Stadtplanung und Landschaftsarchitektur. Stadt und Grün – Das Gartenamt 59(12):17–22

Cervinka R, Höltge J, Pirgie L, Schwab M, Sudkamp J, Haluza D, Arnberger A, Eder R, Ebenberger M (2014) Zur Gesundheitswirkung von Waldlandschaften. Bericht 147/2014. Bundesforschungs- und Ausbildungszentrum für Wald, Naturgefahren und Landschaft, Wien

Chun MH, Chang MC, Lee SJ (2017) The effects of forest therapy on depression and anxiety in patients with chronic stroke. Int J Neurosci 127:199–203

Cimprich B, Ronis DL (2003) An environmental intervention to restore attention in women with newly diagnosed breast cancer. Cancer Nurs 26:284–292

Cohen S, Alper CM, Doyle WJ, Treanor JJ, Turner RB (2006) Positive emotional style predicts resistance to illness after experimental exposure to rhinovirus or influenza A virus. Psychosom Med 68:809–815

Diezemann A (2011) Entspannungsverfahren bei chronischem Schmerz. Schmerz 25:445–453

Dolling A, Nilsson H, Lundell Y (2017) Stress recovery in forest or handicraft environments – an intervention study. Urban For Urban Green 27:162–172

Donovan GH, Butry DT, Michael YL, Prestemon JP, Liebhold AM, Gatziolis D, Mao MY (2013) The relationship between trees and human health: evidence from the spread of the emerald ash borer. Am J Prev Med 44:139–145

Engemann K, Bøcker Pedersen C, Arge L, Tsirogiannis C, Mortensen PB, Svenning JC (2019) Residential green space in childhood is associated with lower risk of psychiatric disorders from adolescence into adulthood. Proc Natl Acad Sci U S A 116:5188–5193

Fessler N (2006) Entspannungsfähigkeit. In: Bös K, Brehm W (eds) Handbuch Gesundheitssport. Hofmann, Schorndorf

Flandroy L, Poutahidis T, Berg G, Clarke G, Dao MC, Decaestecker E, Furman E, Haahtela T, Massart S, Plovier H, Sanz Y, Rook G (2018) The impact of human activities and lifestyles on the interlinked microbiota and health of humans and of ecosystems. Sci Total Environ 15:1018–1038

Han JW, Choi H, Jeon YH, Yoon CH, Woo JM, Kim W (2016) The effects of forest therapy on coping with chronic widespread pain: physiological and psychological differences between participants in a forest therapy programme and a control group. Int J Environ Res Public Health 13:255

Hansen MM, Jones R, Tocchini K (2017) Shinrin-Yoku (forest bathing) and nature therapy: a state-of-the-art review. Int J Environ Res Public Health 14:851

Hanski C, Hertzen LV, Fyhrquist N, Koskinen K, Torppa K, Laatikainen T, Karisola P, Auvinen P, Paulin L, Mäkelä MJ, Vartiainen E, Kosunen TU, Alenius H, Haahtela T (2012) Biodiversity, human microbiota, and allergy. Proc Natl Acad Sci 109:8334–8339

Hapke U, Maske UE, Scheidt-Nave C, Bode L, Schlack R, Busch MA (2013) Chronischer Stress bei Erwachsenen in Deutschland – Ergebnisse der Studie zur Gesundheit Erwachsener in Deutschland (DEGS1). Bundesgesundheitsblatt 56:749–754

Hassan A, Tao J, Li G, Jiang M, Aii L, Zongfang ZL, Qibing C (2018) Effects of walking in bamboo forest and city environments on brainwave activity in young adults. Evid Based Complement Alternat Med 2018:9653857

Hunziker M, Lindern EV, Bauer N, Frick J (2012) Das Verhältnis der Schweizer Bevölkerung zum Wald. In: Eidgenössische Forschungsanstalt für Wald, Schnee und Landschaft (Ed) Waldmonitoring soziokulturell: Weiterentwicklung und zweite Erhebung – WaMos 2. Report, pp 1–182

Ideno Y, Hayashi K, Abe Y, Ueda K, Iso H, Noda M, Lee JS, Suzuki S (2017) Blood pressure-lowering effect of Shinrin-yoku (Forest bathing): a systematic review and meta-analysis. BMC Complement Altern Med 17:409

Im SG, Choi H, Jeon YH, Song MK, Kim W, Woo JM (2016) Comparison of effect of two-hour exposure to forest and urban environments on cytokine, anti-oxidant, and stress levels in young adults. Int J Environ Res Public Health 13:625

Jia BB, Yang ZX, Mao GX, Lyu Y, Wen XL, Xu WH, Lyu Xiao L, Cao YB, Wang GF (2016) Health ffeect of forest bathing trip on elderly patients with chronic obstructive pulmonary disease. Biomed Environ Sci 29:212–218

Kaiserbäder Insel Usedom (2018) Pilotstudie im Heilwald Heringsdorf. https://www.heilwald-heringsdorf.de/Indikation-Heilung/COPD-Pilotstudie. Accessed 12 Dec 2018

Kang B, Kim T, Kim MJ, Lee KH, Choi S, Lee DH, Kim HR, Jun B, Park SY, Lee SJ, Park SB (2015) Relief of chronic posterior neck pain depending on the type of forest therapy: comparison of the therapeutic effect of forest bathing alone versus forest bathing with exercise. Ann Rehabil Med 39:957–963

Kaplan S (1995) The restorative benefits of nature: toward an integrative framework. J Environ Psychol 15:169–182

Kaplan R, Kaplan S (1989) The experience of nature. A psychological perspective. New York, Cambridge University Press

Karjalainen E, Sarjala T, Raitio H (2010) Promoting human health through forests: overview and major challenges. Environ Health Prev Med 15:1–8

Kawada T, Li Q, Nakadai A, Inagaki H, Katsumata M, Shimizu T, Hirata Y, Hirata K, Suzuki H (2012) Effect of forest bathing on sleep and physical activity. In: Li Q (ed) Forest medicine. Nova Science Publishers, New York

Kim W, Lim SK, Chung EJ, Woo JM (2009) The effect of cognitive behavior therapy-based psychotherapy applied in a forest environment on physiological changes and remission of major depressive disorder. Psychiatry Investig 6:245–254

Kim BJ, Jeong H, Park S, Lee S (2015) Forest adjuvant anti-cancer therapy to enhance natural cytotoxicity in urban women with breast cancer: a preliminary prospective interventional study. Eur J Integr Med 7:474–478

Korpela KM, Pasanen T, Repo V, Hartig T, Staats H, Mason M, Alves S, Fornara F, Marks T, Saini S, Scopelliti M, Soares AL, Stigsdotter UK, Ward Thompson C (2018) Environmental strategies of affect regulation and their associations with subjective well-being. Front Psychol 9:562

Kuchma VR, Sukhareva LM, Makarova A (2008) Scientific bases of the improvement of and planting of trees and bushes in the playgrounds of outbuilding areas. (Russian language). Gig Sanit 1:51–55

Kühn S, Düze S, Eibich P, Krekel C, Wüstemann H, Kolbe J, Martensson J, Goebel J, Gallinat J, Wagner GG, Lindenberger U (2017) In search of features that constitute an "enriched environment" in humans: associations between geographical properties and brain structure. Nat Sci Rep 7(11):920

Kuo FE, Faber Taylor A (2004) A potential natural treatment for attention-deficit/hyperactivity disorder: evidence from a national study. Am J Public Health 94:1580–1586

Lee JY, Lee DC (2014) Cardiac and pulmonary benefits of forest walking versus city walking in elderly women: a randomised, controlled, open-label trial. Eur J Integr Med 6:5–11

Lee I, Choi H, Bang KS, Kim S, Song M, Lee B (2017) Effect of forest therapy on depressive symptoms among adults: a systematic review. Int J Environ Res Public Health 14:321

Li Q (2017) Shinrin-yoku: the art and science of forest bathing. Penguin Random House, London

Li Q, Morimoto K, Nakadai A, Inagaki H, Katsumata M, Shimizu T, Hirata Y, Hirata K, Suzuki H, Miyazaki Y, Kagawa T, Koyama Y, Ohira T, Takayama N, Krensky AM, Kawada T (2007) Forest bathing enhances human natural killer activity and expression of anti-cancer proteins. Int J Immunopathol Pharmacol 20:3–8

Li Q, Morimoto K, Kobayashi M, Inagaki H, Katsumata M, Hirata Y, Hirata K, Shimizu T, Li YJ, Wakayama Y, Kawada T, Ohira T, Takayama N, Kagawa T, Miyazaki Y (2008a) A forest bathing trip increases human natural killer activity and expression of anti-cancer proteins in female subjects. J Biol Regul Homeost Agents 22:45–55

Li Q, Morimoto K, Kobayashi M, Inagaki H, Katsumata M, Hirata Y, Hirata K, Suzuki H, Li YJ, Wakayama Y, Kawada T, Park BJ, Ohira T, Matsui N, Kagawa T, Miyazaki Y, Krensky AM (2008b) Visiting a forest, but not a city, increases human natural killer activity and expression of anti-cancer proteins. Int J Immunopathol Pharmacol 21:117–127

Li Q, Kobayashi M, Inagaki H, Hirata Y, Li YJ, Hirata K, Shimizu T, Suzuki H, Katsumata M, Wakayama Y, Kawada T, Ohira T, Matsui N, Kagawa T (2010) A day trip to a forest park increases human natural killer activity and the expression of anti-cancer proteins in male subjects. J Biol Regul Homeost Agents 24:157–165

Li Q, Kobayashi M, Kawada T (2012) Effect of forest coverage on standardized mortality ratios of cancers in Japan. In: Li Q (ed) Forest medicine. Nova Science Publishers, New York

Li D, Larsen L, Yang Y, Wang L, Zhai Y, Sullivan WC (2019) Exposure to nature for children with autism spectrum disorder: benefits, caveats, and barriers. Health Place 55:71–78

Maas J, Verheij RA, Groenewegen PP, De Vries S, Spreeuwenberg P (2006) Green space, urbanity, and health: how strong is the relation? J Epidemiol Community 60:587–592

Mao GX, Cao YB, Lan XG, He ZH, Chen ZM, Wang YZ, Hu XL, Lv YD, Wang GF, Yan J (2012a) Therapeutic effect of forest bathing on human hypertension in the elderly. J Cardiol 60:495–502

Mao GX, Lan XG, Cao YB, Chen ZM, He ZH, Lv YD, Wang YZ, Hu XL, Wang GF, Yan J (2012b) Effects of short-term forest bathing on human health in a broad-leaved evergreen forest in Zhejiang Province, China. Biomed Environ Sci 25:317–324

Mao GX, Cao YB, Yang Y, Chen ZM, Dong JH, Chen SS, Wu Q, Lyu XL, Jia BB, Yan J, Wang GF (2018) Additive benefits of twice forest bathing trips in elderly patients with chronic heart failure. Biomed Environ Sci 31:159–162

Matsunaga K, Park BJ, Kobayashi H, Miyazaki Y (2011) Physiologically relaxing effect of a hospital rooftop forest on older women requiring care. JAGS 59:2162

Meyer K, Bürger-Arndt R (2014) How forests foster human health – present state of research-based knowledge (in the field of forests and human health). Int For Rev 16:421–446

Mitchell R, Popham F (2008) Effect of exposure to natural environment on health inequalities: an observational population study. Lancet 372:1655–1660

Morita E, Fukuda S, Nagano J, Hamajima N, Yamamoto H, Iwai Y, Nakashima T, Ohira H, Shirakawa T (2007) Psychological effects of forest environments on healthy adults: Shinrin-yoku (forest-air bathing, walking) as a possible method of stress reduction. Public Health 121:54–63

Morita E, Naito M, Hishida A, Wakai K, Mori A, Asai Y, Okada R, Kawai S, Hamajima N (2011a) No association between the frequency of forest walking and blood pressure levels or the prevalence of hypertension in a cross-sectional study of a Japanese population. Environ Health Prev Med 16:299–306

Morita E, Imai M, Okawa M, Miyaura T, Miyazaki S (2011b) A before and after comparison of the effects of forest walking on the sleep of a community-based sample of people with sleep complaints. BioPsychoSocial Med 5:13

Nilsson K, Sangster M, Gallis C, Hartig T, de Vries S, Seeland K, Schipperijn J (eds) (2011) Forests, trees and human health. Springer, New York/Dordrecht/ Heidelberg/London

O'Brien L, Morris J, Stewart A (2012) Forest research exploring relationships between peri-urban woodlands and people's health and well-being. Social and Economic Research Group of the Research Agency of the Forestry Commission. Crown Publisher, London

Oh B, Lee KJ, Zaslawski C, Yeung A, Rosenthal D, Larkey L, Back M (2017) Health and well-being benefits of spending time in forests: systematic review. Environ Health Prev Med 22:71

Ohe Y (2017) Evaluating the relaxation effects of emerging forest-therapy tourism: a multidisciplinary approach. Tour Manag 62:322–334

Ohira H, Takagi S, Masui K, Oishi M, Obata A (1999) Effect of Shinrin-yoku (forest-air bathing and walking): on mental and physical health (in Japanese). Bull Tokai Women's Collect 19:217–232

Orr N, Wagstaffe A, Briscoe S, Garside R (2016) How do older people describe their sensory experiences of the natural world? A systematic review of the qualitative evidence. BMC Geriatr 16:116

Park BJ, Tsunetsugu Y, Kasetani T, Hirano H, Kagawa T, Sato M, Miyazaki Y (2007) Physiological effects of Shinrin-yoku (taking in the atmosphere of the forest)-using salivary cortisol and cerebral activity as indicators. J Physiol Anthropol 26:123–128

Park BJ, Tsunetsugu Y, Kasetani T, Kagawa T, Miyazaki Y (2010) The physiological effects of Shinrin-yoku (taking in the forest atmosphere or forest bathing): evidence from field experiments in 24 forests across Japan. Environ Health Prev Med 15:18–26

Park BJ, Tsunetsugu Y, Lee J, Kagawa T, Miyazaki Y (2011) Effect of the forest environment on physiological relaxation using the results of field tests at 35 sites throughout Japan. In: Li Q (ed) Forest medicine. Nova Science Publishers, New York

Rook GA (2013) Regulation of the immune system by biodiversity from the natural environment: an ecosystem service essential to health. Proc Natl Acad Sci U S A:110, 18.360–18.367

Roovers P, Hermy M, Gulnick H (2002) A survey of recreation interests in urban forests, the influence of travel distance. In: Arnberger A, Brandenburg C, Muhar A (eds) Monitoring and management of visitor flows in recreational and protected areas. Conference Proceedings, Wien, pp 277–283

Seo SC, Park SJ, Park CW, Yoon WS, Choung JT, Yoo Y (2015) Clinical and immunological effects of a forest trip in children with asthma and atopic dermatitis. Iran J Allergy Asthma Immunol 14:28–36

Shin WS, Yeoun PS, Yoo RW, Shin CS (2010) Forest experience and psychological health benefits: the state of the art and future prospect in Korea. Environ Health Prev Med 15:38–47

Shin WS, Shin CS, Yeoun PS (2012) The influence of forest therapy camp on depression in alcoholics. Environ Health Prev Med 17:73–76

Sivarajah S, Smith SM, Thomas SC (2018) Tree cover and species composition effects on academic performance of primary school students. PLoS One 13:e0193254

Sluiter JK, van der Beek AJ, Frings-Dresen MH (1999) The influence of work characteristics on the need for recovery and experienced health: a study on coach drivers. Ergonomics 42:573–583

Song C, Ikei H, Lee J, Park BJ, Kagawa T, Miyazaki Y (2013) Individual differences in the physiological effects of forest therapy based on Type A and Type B behavior patterns. J Physiol Anthropol 32:14

Song C, Ikei H, Kobayashi M, Miura T, Taue M, Kagawa T, Li Q, Kumeda S, Imai M, Miyazaki Y (2015) Effect of forest walking on autonomic nervous system activity in middle-aged hypertensive individuals. Int J Environ Res Public Health 12:2687–2699

Song C, Ikei H, Miyazaki Y (2018) Physiological effects of visual stimulation with forest imagery. Int J Environ Res Public Health 15:213

Sonntag-Öström E, Nordin M, Järvholm LS, Lundell Y, Brännström R, Dolling A (2011) Can the boreal forest be used for rehabilitation and recovery from stress-related exhaustion? A pilot study. Scand J For Res 26:245–256

Stark JH, Neckerman K, Lovasi GS, Quinn J, Weiss CC, Bader MDM, Konto K, Harris TG, Rundle A (2014) The impact of neighborhood park access and quality on body mass index among adults in New York City. Prev Med 64:63–68

Stigsdotter UK, Corazon SS, Sidenius U, Kristiansen J, Grahn P (2017) It is not all bad for the grey city – a crossover study on physiological and psychological restoration in a forest and an urban environment. Health Place 46:145–154

Sulander T, Karvinen E, Holopainen M (2016) Urban green space visits and mortality among older adults. Epidemiology 27. https://doi.org/10.1097/EDE.0000000000000511

Tsao TM, Tsai MJ, Wang YN, Lin HL, Wu CF, Hwang JS, Hsu SHJ, Chao H, Chuang KJ, Chou CCK, Su TC (2014) The health effects of a forest environment on subclinical cardiovascular disease and heath-related quality of life. PLoS One 9:e103231

Tsunetsugu Y, Park BJ, Miyazaki Y (2010) Trends in research related to "Shinrin-yoku" (taking in the forest atmosphere or forest bathing) in Japan. Environ Health Prev Med 15:27

Ulrich RS (1979) Visual landscapes and psychological well-being. Landsc Res 4:17–23

Vaitl D (2009) Neurobiologische Grundlagen der Entspannungsverfahren. In: Petermann F, Vaitl D (eds) . Entspannungsverfahren. Das Praxishandbuch. Beltz, Weinheim

van Hooff ML, Geurts SA, Kompier MA, Taris TW (2007) Workdays, in-between workdays and the weekend: a diary study on effort and recovery. Int Arch Occup Environ Health 80:599–613

Vocks E, Busch R, Fröhlich C, Borelli S, Mayer H, Ring J (2001) Influence of weather and climate on subjective symptom intensity in atopic eczema. Int J Biometeorol 45:27–33

Von Mutius E (2019) Die Rolle des Umweltmikrobioms in der Asthma- und Allergieentstehung. In: Bayerische Akademie der Wissenschaften (ed) Die unbekannte Welt der Mikrobiome, Bd 47. Dr. Friedrich Pfeil, München

Whear R, Coon JT, Bethel A, Abbott R, Stein K, Garside R (2014) What is the impact of using outdoor spaces such as gardens on the physical and mental well-being of those with dementia? A systematic review of quantitative and qualitative evidence. J Am Med Dir Assoc 15:697–705

White MP, Alcock I, Grellier J, Wheeler BW, Hartig T, Warber SL, Bone A, Depledge MH, Fleming LE (2019) Spending at least 120 minutes a week in nature is associated with good health and wellbeing. Nat Sci Rep 9:7730

Wu J, Jackson L (2017) Inverse relationship between urban green space and childhood autism in California elementary school districts. Environ Int 107:140–146

Wu J, Rappazzo KM, Simpson RJ Jr, Joodi G, Pursell IW, Mounsey JP, Cascio WE, Jackson LE (2018) Exploring links between greenspace and sudden unexpected death: spatial analysis. Environ Int 113:114–121

Wyles KJ, White MP, Hattam C, Pahl S, King H, Austen M (2017) Are some natural environments more psychologically beneficial than others? The importance of type and quality on connectedness to nature and psychological restoration. Environ Behav 51:111–143

Yatsunenko T, Rey FE, Manary MJ, Trehan I, Dominguez-Bello MG, Contreras M, Magris M, Hidalgo G, Baldassano RN, Anokhin AP, Heath AC, Warner B, Reeder J, Kuczynski J, Caporaso JG, Lozupone CA, Lauber C, Clemente JC, Knights D, Knight R, Gordon JI (2012) Human gut microbiome viewed across age and geography. Nature 486(7402):222–227

Yu CP, Lin CM, Tsai MJ, Tsai YC, Chen CY (2017) Effects of short forest bathing programme on autonomic nervous system activity and mood states in middle-aged and elderly individuals. Int J Environ Res Public Health 14:897

Zundel R, Völksen G (2002) Ergebnisse der Walderholungsforschung. Eine verglei-chende Darstellung deutschsprachiger Untersuchungen. Universität Göttingen, Göttingen

5

How to Discover and Utilise the Forest for Your Health

Summary

This practically-oriented chapter shows the most important characteristics of a forest for Shinrin-Yoku and deals with the development of cure and healing forests as well as with the special professional qualification courses to become a forest health trainer and forest therapist. Health promotion and prevention as important modules are defined and examples of implementation in the forest are presented. Mindfulness, body-mind procedures and other naturopathic techniques that can be applied in the forest either as a focus or as an accompanying intervention, are explained from a scientific point of view. Finally, it is shown that forests cannot simply be used commercially, but that certain guidelines must be observed.

5.1 Which Forest Is Suitable for Forest Therapy?

Forests are perceived differently depending on individual landscape preferences. Nevertheless, there are generalisable preferences and limitations in the assessment of forests and the question of the optimal forest.

The *mixed* coniferous and deciduous forest is considered the most popular forest structure. A mixed forest changes in the year in terms of its forms, but above all in terms of colours and light effects, and is regarded as a guarantor of a certain naturalness as well as species and animal richness. The mixed forest is often described with attributes such as friendly, natural and healthy,

© Springer-Verlag GmbH Germany, part of Springer Nature 2022
A. Schuh, G. Immich, *Forest Therapy - The Potential of the Forest for Your Health*,
https://doi.org/10.1007/978-3-662-64280-1_5

whereas a pure coniferous forest often receives negative evaluations (monoculture, dense, uniform stocking and size, shady, dark) (Braun 2000).

In addition to the key aesthetic elements (see Sect. 3.3), there are important characteristics of a forest and its atmosphere that should be taken into account when using it for forest bathing and forest therapy (Table 5.1).

The *density* of the forest is extremely important for well-being (Takayama et al. 2017): In one study, the preferences between a dense, impenetrable and a sparser coniferous forest were examined. The young students surveyed felt more comfortable in the light coniferous forest and preferred it. The two forests differ in that sunlight penetrates more in the light coniferous forest and it is about twice as bright as in the dense forest. The dense coniferous forest, which seemed more "natural", was nevertheless rated as "darker, more closed, rather unpleasant, not inviting, chaotic and rather unhealthier". In contrast, the sparser coniferous forest was described as "managed, more beautiful, more refreshing". The mood-lifting effect of the forest is thus particularly influenced by the light conditions in the forest. A translucent forest can improve mood when sunlight falls through the leaves, creating a pleasant atmosphere. White birch trunks also enhanced the light effect. Healthy horticulture students who spent an hour each in birch, maple, or oak forest described the birch forest they visited as being more light-filled because it allowed the sun's rays to penetrate more clearly and enhanced the contrast between the white

Table 5.1 Important criteria for the use of a forest for forest bathing. For therapeutic use, further add-ons are required to the special needs of different patients

Density of the forest	Light forest: Lighter, less constricting or oppressive than darker, denser forest.
Special features (tree majesties or groupings)	Old and beautiful trees
Biodiversity	Different tree species and plant vegetation
Colour change	Play of colours, light-dark, different shades of green
Different vegetation	Different shapes, heights of the stand, forest edge design
Stock structure	The alternation between sparse and dense vegetation
Stock openings	Clearings, forest meadows, aisles
Variety	Natural forest, no monotony, curved, hidden paths
Water areas (blue space)	Rivers, streams, lakes
Forest floor	Natural forest floor, soft and diverse
Forest typical silence	Lively sounds of nature, typical forest "silence", important criterion!
Forest smell	Different sensory olfactory inspirations

trunk and coloured foliage. In this forest, the participants felt slightly more comfortable and experienced less anxiety than in the maple or oak forest (Guan et al. 2017).

The *age and beauty* of trees also represent an essential criterion for the selection of a Shinrin-Yoku forest. The outer form of a tree and its crown density lead to different individual well-being preferences. Among the German population, large, sprawling deciduous trees are particularly popular (Hofmann et al. 2017). Old trees are often particularly strikingly shaped and impress with their size and span. The old "tree personalities"—especially when they are free-standing (solitaires)—have a powerful aura and convey respect for nature ("awe"). In their presence, everyday problems can lose their significance. For this reason, such striking solitary trees are often chosen as favourite places within a forest. They can also serve as recognition features or landmarks in the forest.

A variety of *different tree and plant species* contributes to the perception that the forest is healthy and pristine, which is often equated with healthy biodiversity. More than three-quarters of all Germans value the forest for its vitality and diversity (Kleinhückelkotten and Neitzke 2010). However, stand density and vegetation are limiting factors, because if they are very pronounced, the visual depth effect of the forest is limited.

The *richness of colour* in the forests is perceived as pleasant. The green colour (see Sect. 3.2) is a sign of nature. Bright green is associated with growth and life. The shades and gradations of green in the leaves and needles of trees and plants convey different spatial depth effects, which also enables different exercises. Colourful blossoms within the greenery of the forest indicate a varied, species-rich natural landscape. The colourful leaves of the deciduous trees in autumn and the autumn foliage delight us—a large proportion of people admire the richness of colour in the autumnal forest.

Different shapes and heights of leaves, plants and trees also contribute to, for example, mindfulness-oriented forest bathing units. In addition to the unique diverse leaf shapes of deciduous trees as well as the branching of coniferous trees, the symmetrical growth forms of trees are an extremely appealing element of the forest. Different tall trees draw different depth effects of the forest. A mixture of young small trees to large old or dead trees with abundant regrowth convey an image of naturalness and vitality, but also of transience and can stimulate reflection or reorientation. Furthermore, light treetops create manifold light and shadow effects. Whereas a closed canopy makes the forest dark but is appreciated as a source of shade in summer. In addition, *different structures* in the forest and the alternation between harmony and disharmony, for example through well-kept sections and opaque growth, light and shadow, as well as narrowness and expanse, appeal to us. During forest therapy, the participants' interests can be focused on the different structures. Quiet corners or fallen trees complement the forest image in this sense, as do beautiful *views* in the form of forest clearings, aisles and forest meadows, which have a special significance in the forest. One can rest there, consciously perceive the forest and enjoy the peace, perhaps even warm up in the sun. An open view of a variety of tree and plant species or even over the treetops into the valley opens up a new perspective for the forest bathing participants. A *varied* forest scenery, which is hilly, appeals to us. For example, a dark forest scene may be in the foreground, but a sunny clearing opens up in the background. Such scenery is known in American parlance as the "mystery effect" and is an excellent way to use a forest. They also include *winding narrow forest paths*. They are considered to be attractive because they provide only a limited view of the next forest areas and thus offer unsuspected vistas. *Natural bodies of water* such as streams, rivers, waterfalls or small ponds also provide new insights and views. *Soft forest floors* with different carpet-like structures of mosses, leaves or coniferous forest litter offer wonderful possibilities for Tai Chi or Qigong (see Sect. 5.4). Also walking on a mossy floor, for example during a walking meditation (5.4), is like floating along. The key aesthetic elements of the forest-typical *silence, nature sounds, the typical smell of the forest,* and *fresh air* (see Sect. 3.2) must be present. If the forest tranquillity is interrupted by man-made soundscapes and these are perceived as disturbing, this massively limits the effects of forest bathing, as does bad air caused by forestry work or a nearby road. The forest boundaries should be loose and also allow a view out of the forest.

Forests with a large *proportion* of deadwood and many dead trees are not suitable for forest therapy, because they do not correspond to a feel-good space and are rather perceived as stressful. A walk in a well-kept forest with a low proportion of deadwood and reduced vegetation density is perceived as more pleasant than walking in an overgrown forest (Bauer et al. 2016).

The suitability of a forest for forest therapy is to a large extent also based on its *accessibility* and the special natural features. For stressed urban people, forest areas close to the city and in the inner city are almost more important than remote recreational forests. Quick accessibility, if possible still by bicycle, is important. In the "Urban Forest 2050" project of the Technical University of Munich, a maximum walking distance of about 300 m for visiting the forest was determined—if the forest is further away, it is less visited (Lupp et al. 2017). Poor public transport connections also lead to people staying away. In addition, recreational visits to the forest have become shorter and shorter in recent years, usually lasting only about 90 min (Weitmann and Korny 2014).

The forest that meets German requirements and is suitable for Shinrin-Yoku and forest therapy is thus a mixed forest with a "feel-good atmosphere".

5.2 Cure and Healing Forests, Forest Health Trainers and Forest Therapists

5.2.1 Conditions and Structures of Cure and Healing Forests

Several European countries now have cure or healing forests. In Germany, Mecklenburg-Western Pomerania takes a pioneering position. It is the first federal state in which, in addition to a useful, protective and recreational function, the health function in the form of cure and healing forests was anchored in the State Forest Act (§ 22). In Heringsdorf on the island of Usedom, the first cure and healing forest was opened in 2017, which is primarily aimed at rehabilitation patients, the chronically ill and senior citizens, but is also open to the healthy population and guests.

In the meantime, other German federal states are working on the implementation of cure and healing forests.

Anyone wishing to operate a cure and healing forest needs a managed forest area suitable for this purpose. The advantage of managed forests is the use of existing paths, the timely elimination of typical forest hazards and possible optimisation of certain forest areas for targeted therapeutic use.

The specific requirements for natural forest conditions are described in a new catalogue of criteria for the Bavarian cure and healing forests (Immich et al. in pep.). It is based on an earlier assessment of the criteria of cure and healing forests for Mecklenburg-Western Pomerania (Schuh and Immich 2013), which is now being adapted to the different conditions throughout the state and the current state of knowledge and requirements.

Accordingly, the *cure forest* represents an environment for health promotion and prevention and is—as the name suggests—preferably located in a health resort. The cure forest should be a well-maintained and near-natural forest, whose characteristics are suitable for Shinrin-Yoku (see Sect. 5.1), and have a corresponding (infra)structural orientation. The focus is on forest experiences, peace and security in the forest, but also on relaxation and mood enhancement. Therapeutic hiking with and without accompaniment in the clean forest air should also be possible in the cure forest. The participants are accompanied and guided by forest health trainers (see below). The structures, i.e. the design of a cure forest, are thus already subject to special requirements. The general rest and recreation function must be underlined. The forest should contain areas for relaxation, exercise, seating and resting facilities. Signage, parking facilities nearby, an appropriate entrance area with toilets and cloakrooms are favourable. In addition to the structures listed above, the health-promoting effects of the forest climate with the entire forest atmosphere are most important in the cure forest.

The *healing forest* can be understood as a "treatment room" and is also located in a health resort or spa and/or near a rehabilitation clinic. It should be accessible primarily only to the target group and contain facilities that enable treatment or rehabilitation measures to be carried out there under professional guidance. Healing forests should also be accessible to people with disabilities. Thus, barrier-free transport connections are essential, as is the existence of barrier-free paths in the forest. Wheelchair users require a different path design than blind people. Hazards due to different use of the paths must be excluded.

Overall, the designation of healing forests places considerable demands on planning. To live up to its claim as the highest "predicate" in forest therapy, a healing forest should comprise a rather small, but high-quality equipped forest or forest section. The healing forest should represent a self-contained unit, i.e. a therapeutic setting, and should be distinguished from the cure forest by increased infrastructural requirements.

In the healing forests, patients and spa guests should also be guided in prevention, but mainly in therapeutic or rehabilitative measures. This requires specialist professional guidance (physiotherapist, sports therapist, climatotherapist) for groups and individuals as well as individual and group therapies. These tasks can also be taken over by a special "forest therapist" (see below).

During forest therapy measures, the participants' need for privacy must be guaranteed and disturbances by uninvolved third parties must be excluded or kept as low as possible. For this reason, it is favourable if a healing forest in which sick people or people with impairments are treated is attached to a clinic and, if possible, is used exclusively by the clinic.

However, when using public forests as cure or healing forests, the possibility of disturbance by others is quite relevant, and at least some protection from noisy visitors must be ensured. Forest bathers and uninvolved forest visitors should be directed through appropriate *visitor management to minimise interference with forest therapy activities.* The topography of the terrain, special features of the vegetation (thickets, etc.) and other natural barriers can be used to separate areas used for therapeutic purposes, at least visually, and to provide natural privacy from prying eyes. In this way, spa guests, patients and therapists can be offered at least a certain minimum of privacy.

Another important aspect of visitor management is to minimise the potential danger posed by other forest visitors and recreational sportsmen (cyclists etc.) to participants in forest therapy programmes, and especially to people with limited mobility.

For the establishment or designation of a cure and healing forest, numerous *legal requirements* and restrictions must also be observed. More details of the German legislation are given in Sect. 5.5.

5.2.2 Prerequisites for Forest Health Trainers and Forest Therapists

Shinrin-Yoku should be instructed and performed with the guests or patients by specially trained personnel.

However, a large field of Shinrin Yoku guides, forest bathing guides, nature coaches or mindfulness trainers in the forest has already formed worldwide. Since there are no uniformly valid definitions or training standards, it is not easy for potential customers/interested parties to get an overview.

If only health promotion and (primary) preventive interventions (see Sect. 5.3) are undertaken, the German *forest health trainers,* for example, who are called "Shinrin-Yoku Guides" in forest bathing in Japan, are suitable. They may come from professional groups in the health and wellness sector or the "green" professions. These and also "only" interested health-conscious people can be trained in a special advanced professional qualification course to become certified Forest Health Trainers (organizer: Chair of Public Health and Health Services Research (IBE) of the Ludwig-Maximilians-University Munich in cooperation with the Competence Centre of Forest Medicine and Nature Therapy, Medical Society for Preventive Medicine and Natural Remedies, Kneippärztebund e.V.). Through this training, participants are enabled to activate the individual body's ordering and healing powers of people with Shinrin-Yoku in the context of health promotion and general prevention. They learn to carry out relaxation exercises and mindfulness procedures with guests (see Sect. 5.4.1), they instruct them in fresh-air rest cures and light climatic terrain treatment (see Sect. 5.4.2) as well as in further preventive methods (such as breathing exercises or Kneipp water applications).

Forest therapists—analogous to the Japanese "Forest Therapist"—are in demand when health disorders are already present or special indications need to be treated. These include not only physical ailments, but also severe stress with corresponding manifestations such as burn-out syndrome or depression. The prerequisite for this profession is a medical background, i.e. a solid therapeutic background, at least as a physiotherapist or similar. Depending on the severity of the illness, doctors or psychologists should also take on this task and complete further training as forest therapists. Here, too, the Chair of Public Health and Health Services Research (IBE) of the Ludwig-Maximilians-University of Munich, Germany, together with the Medical Society for Preventive Medicine and Natural Remedies, Kneippärztebund e.V., will set up a corresponding professional qualification course to become a certified forest therapist.

5.3   Health Promotion in the Forest

Health promotion and preventive interventions are intended to strengthen health at an early stage to prevent the development of risk factors and diseases.

Health promotion focuses on the consolidation of health resources and anchoring coping strategies, especially in the personal and social environment. Health promotion is thus aimed at people who want to shape their lifestyles in a health-conscious way so that they can continue to lead a healthy life. Health promotion is one of the important goals of Shinrin-Yoku.

Prevention (health care) includes the targeted avoidance of disease-causing behavior as well as of already existing risk factors and their manifestation. Preventing further progression of a disease (see below) is also part of prevention in the broadest sense. A distinction is made between three levels of prevention:

Primary prevention is aimed at healthy people who already have identifiable risk factors. The aim is to maintain health and prevent disease by minimising or eliminating known or existing causes of disease, such as obesity or physical inactivity (Franzkowiak 2018). Lifestyle changes are often considered for this purpose.

Secondary prevention, on the other hand, is intended to prevent already existing health disorders (such as elevated blood sugar) from triggering acute illnesses (such as heart attacks) or manifesting themselves in chronic diseases. The aim of secondary prevention is thus the early detection of disease with a reduction or avoidance of exacerbation and its chronification (ibid.).

Tertiary prevention corresponds to rehabilitation, i.e. treatment after an acute illness or in the case of a chronic illness, aimed at preventing a permanent loss of function or restriction with reduced participation (ibid.).

Shinrin-Yoku with its different methods is until today mainly health-promoting as well as primary preventive oriented, but can also be carried out in the field of secondary prevention and as an accompanying rehabilitation intervention.

Health-promoting programmes as well as primary prevention in the forest are based on the findings of medical climatology, naturopathic therapies, recreation and stress research as well as ecopsychological knowledge and can be offered and guided by specially trained "Forest Health Trainers". Secondary preventive or rehabilitative interventions during forest therapy should be guided by appropriately trained medical professionals such as "Forest Therapists " (see Sect. 5.2).

Depending on the target group, *different concepts for health promotion or prevention* can be implemented in the forest. For a good recovery effect, a balanced alternation of stress and relief (change in the level of demand), as well as activation and deactivation (change in the level of activation), is necessary (Allmer 1996). In the case of excessive demands due to exhaustion (or illness), it is important to recharge one's batteries, rest and thus counteract further resource depletion. Especially in the case of stress, the excessive activation level must be lowered to release tension/cramps and come to rest. In contrast to this, mental as well as physical activity is required in the case of underload. In the case of a strain due to mental over-saturation, meaningful activity creates a balance. Thus, a rough distinction can be made between two recovery strategies (Allmer 1996): a programme for people with an overload problem and a programme for people who feel constantly under-challenged. Finally, these preventive forest programmes can be individually adapted in a more differentiated way according to the respective forms of stress.

Examples
Stressed, mentally distressed individuals:
Psychologically stressed persons often feel that they can no longer cope with a situation or requirement; it is difficult or completely impossible to switch off from stressful situations or responsibilities. Physically, the stress manifests itself in muscular tension, among other things. The recovery strategy aims to reduce the excessive activation level through a guided stay in the forest and thus to normalise and release tensions/cramps (Allmer 1996).

Therefore, it makes sense for stressed persons to initiate recovery processes by switching from the cognitive functional level to the sensory and emotional level. Due to this refocusing or reorientation of perception, mental health (ability to concentrate, alertness) can be restored. Best suited for this purpose are the different sensory exercises that can be performed during Shinrin-Yoku.

Furthermore, procedures or exercises that build up and deepen the quality of connectedness to nature and thus create an emotional connection between man and nature are purposeful. In addition, body-mind techniques and relaxation techniques (see below) are excellent ways to recharge one's batteries in the forest and promote relaxation.

People with symptoms of fatigue due to mental or physical overload:

Physical, but also cognitive exhaustion as a result of excessive demands in everyday life requires a general reduction of demands as a recovery strategy in order not to further minimize the already exhausted resources (Kaiser 2016). The goal is to refuel physical energy resources and regain one's strength to be able to meet future demands. In doing so, forest bathing should be carried out with a reduced, i.e. light, physical and mental energy expenditure. It has also been proven that a light exercise intervention is superior to recovery through rest (Beckmann and Fröhlich 2009). For example, various exercises for sensory perception, mindfulness exercises and decelerating walking or strolling are suitable for this purpose.

People with mental or physical underachievement:

If the daily work routine is monotonous and under challenging, stress occurs due to a lack of cognitive, emotional and physical stimuli and demands. The recovery measure aims to achieve a balancing or stimulating effect through physical activity or new cognitive and emotional stimuli. In this context, the new different stimuli or activities represent a recovery-promoting load and seem to be necessary for a recovery process. For example, imparting specific forest knowledge can provide a knowledge stimulus, or addressing the different sensory qualities during a forest experience can revitalize and deepen body perception. Moderate exercise therapy and well-dosed Kneipp applications in the form of a foot or arm bath also raise the activity level and can be continued at home after forest bathing, as well as Tai Chi exercises that certainly challenge the practitioner in their complexity and can also be adopted in everyday life (see Sect. 5.4). By practising nature connectedness, new emotional aspects can be initiated and deepened.

People with psychic saturation:

The everyday lack of meaningful, satisfying activities leads to increased psychological stress, since one's own needs are negated or cannot be lived out to the full. The recreational measure aims to rediscover the meaningfulness of one's actions in life, i.e. to rediscover and enjoy the individual joy of life by immersing oneself in the forest with all the senses. Likewise, the fact of a stronger connection to nature can be seen as an important emotional factor that has a positive effect on the general well-being and personal satisfaction with life.

When choosing a forest bathing format, however, it is important to bear in mind that excessive demands with fatigue and high-stress levels can lead to profound states of exhaustion in the long term. These can be alleviated somewhat in the short term by "skilfully guided" forest bathing sessions. Nevertheless, such states of exhaustion require a longer-term rest or recovery phase. This should be supported by repeated forest bathing sessions to replenish energy resources more quickly.

In the case of psychological stress due to under challenge, immersion in the atmosphere of the forest breaks through the monotony of everyday life, and new types of stimuli and content, mostly foreign, are immediately received and perceived. The creation of an emotional connection to nature can be helpful as a key element in this process. However, this often requires good and targeted guidance that appeals to the participants.

5.4 Health-Promoting Practices/Applications in the Forest

5.4.1 Mindfulness Procedures, Body-Mind and Relaxation Techniques

"Modern" and easy to apply in the forest are the methods Qigong and Tai Chi, which originate mainly from the Asian region. They are used in forest therapy in Japan, China and Korea. Yoga can also be part of it. Important for forest therapy are also mindfulness exercises to enhance the sensory perception in order to development a connection to nature. The well-known methods such as progressive muscle relaxation or autogenic training are rather less suitable for forest bathing or forest therapy, as they are carried out in a quiet lying position and are only possible on warm days, even if a suitable infrastructure is available.

Body-mind techniques and mindfulness exercises reduce stress levels and lead to sympathetic modulation (Zou et al. 2018). Various studies also indicate that body-mind procedures or relaxation procedures are predominantly suitable for mental stress at work as a targeted and effective recovery procedure. Even sport seems to reduce rumination (the constant circling of thoughts around problems) less effectively than active relaxation techniques (Allmer 1996). Other positive effects include improved concentration, increased self-confidence, sensitization of the body's perceptions, anxiety reduction, and an increase in mood and well-being (Kaiser 2016).

Mindfulness-Based Stress Reduction Programmes

Mindfulness techniques help to better control attention (Esch 2014) by expanding the "flashlight cone of consciousness" and consequently noticing more in and around oneself. Mindfulness practice as a body-mind practise aims to connect psyche, emotion, mind, spirit and body to protect against overload and exhaustion and to strengthen self-efficacy, connectedness and inner satisfaction.

Mindfulness practice enhances body awareness and increases acceptance of one's own body. The goal of mindfulness practice is to improve self-awareness and differentiation of what is important and what is not, as well as a more detached approach to stressful thoughts, emotions and stress. This emotional self-regulation is credited with leading to systematic desensitization to negative emotions and compassion, and increased openness and equanimity. A mindful attitude also affects memory capacity and thus improves learning and retentiveness (Esch 2014).

When mindfulness exercises are carried out in nature (forest), they make it possible to immerse oneself in diverse moods and to enjoy and preserve them in their complex biodiversity. In the process, the positive image of closeness to nature is formed.

There are several types of programmes: Mindfulness-based stress reduction (MBSR), mindfulness-based cognitive therapy (MBCT), dialectical-behavioral therapy (DBT), and acceptance and commitment therapy (ACT).

The best-known method is the mindfulness-based stress reduction programme MBSR. The method originates from Buddhist teachings and Eastern meditation practices and was developed in the 1980s. It involves being intentional/well-intentioned in mindset and activities, relating only to the present moment, and being mindful, open, and non-judgmental of all thoughts/feelings. It is a consciously taken attitude. Thus, self-esteem as a central health resource that protects against overload and exhaustion represents the goal.

The evidence of effectiveness has been confirmed by a large number of meta-analysis (including Khoury et al. 2015). According to this, the mindfulness method MBSR leads to a reduction/improvement of symptoms in anxiety, depression, stress, heart disease, musculoskeletal diseases, cancer, HIV and addiction. MBSR is also part of the German medical guidelines for the treatment of depressive disorders in children/adolescents and in the treatment of unipolar depression in adults. It is a recognized preventive service of the German health insurance according to § 20.

Meditation

For thousands of years, meditation has been a proven and well-known method of bringing peace to the body and mind and counteracting stress and negative emotions. Especially in the Asian tradition, different types of meditation are used in everyday life. Passive meditations such as resting or breathing meditations can be distinguished from active forms such as walking meditation. What they all have in common is a clearly positive relaxation effect, followed by greater emotion control and self-regulation, which have been confirmed by various studies and reviews (including Esch 2014). For mindfulness meditation, for example, positive effects such as the reduction of anxiety, depression, stress, pain, as well as an improvement in mental mood, attention and a higher quality of life have been demonstrated (Goyal et al. 2015).

Meditation can be done in the forest in a simple form as sitting meditation, for example on a tree stump. Sitting meditation involves quiet, relaxed and open perception and taking in the surrounding nature. Walking meditation can also provide new emotions and sensory perceptions in the forest.

Tai Chi Chuan

The literal translation of Tai Chi Chuan is "supreme ultimate fist". The origin lies in China as a martial art. In the Asian philosophical sense and according to Traditional Chinese Medicine, Tai Chi—like Qigong (see below)—promotes the flow of Qi, the life energy. In the western sense, Tai Chi belongs to the body-mind-methods. It reduces stress and increases physical well-being. Its main elements are movement, meditation and deep abdominal breathing. Tai Chi is excellent for forest therapy (3sat 2019). Numerous studies looking at the effects of Tai Chi Chuan. It shows excellent effects in rehabilitation, but also in health promotion and prevention.

The slow movements make the exercises also possible for older people. Improvements in balance have been known for a long time and Tai Chi is used for fall prevention. The general fitness of seniors increases and there are corresponding adaptive reactions in the cardiovascular and the muscular system (Chodzko-Zajko et al. 2009). Age-related sleep disorders (Yeh et al. 2008) are improved, and the psychosocial participation of the elderly is increased by Tai Chi (Huang et al. 2017).

Tai Chi is also suitable for healthy middle-aged and younger people. Countless studies have proven that regular Tai Chi exercises lead to stress reduction and simultaneous reduction of cardiovascular risk factors on all levels in terms of prevention. In addition to improving sleep and mood, it affects mental health and agility (Liu et al. 2018). Other psychological effects such as mood improvement, anxiety reduction, and increased self-assessment have been documented, as well as a positive impact on psychosocial and emotional well-being.

Although slow movements are performed, they require considerable muscle work, especially of the arms and legs, even though squatting position (slightly bent knees). There is an increase in muscular strength and muscular endurance and an increase in overall physical fitness. Thus, a study in which Tai Chi versus walking (12 weeks each) was investigated (Hui et al. 2009) also showed significant and comparable effects on physical performance and muscular fitness, blood sugar levels, resting metabolism and general health.

Tai Chi is therefore a so-called aerobic training with moderate intensity. The power achieved during Tai Chi exercises is equivalent to walking at 6 km/h (Lan et al. 2008) and is thus in the internationally recognised range for moderate endurance training.

In the rehabilitation of existing diseases, various systematic reviews and meta-analysis show the evident effects of regular Tai Chi exercises, for example, in depressive symptoms, coronary heart disease and various diseases of the musculoskeletal system such as rheumatoid arthritis, fibromyalgia, or non-specific chronic back pain: Tai Chi is the best-studied and best-evidenced body-mind method and, from the Asian tradition alone, is excellently suited for use in forest therapy and can be performed in almost any weather.

Qigong

Qigong is also an excellent method for Shinrin-Yoku. It requires no equipment or infrastructure.

Qigong is exercised regularly by millions of Chinese people. In Chinese medicine, a free flow of Qi in the meridians means that body, mind and spirit are in harmony, and that means health. A blocked Qi is said to lead to illness. Qigong is an element of Traditional Chinese Medicine (TCM). It exercises the mind and body simultaneously and can therefore be called a "body-mind" intervention. It is used to treat various chronic diseases and to promote healthy living. A distinction is made between "Medical Qigong", which is done with a TCM doctor, and "Prevention Qigong". The main elements are mind, breath, posture and movement. According to a meta-analysis, Qigong has proven effects in terms of general prevention and secondary prevention (Ng and Tsang 2009). The mechanisms of action are still unclear. Psychophysiological mechanisms that influence the immune system, sympathicotonic and parasympathetic nervous system and hormones can be considered.

For medical Qigong, numerous studies from China show evidence, for example, for the treatment of hypertension, fibromyalgia or Parkinson's disease. In addition, although there are still no clear results, there are indications of a beneficial effect in the prevention of stroke, both for Tai Chi and Qigong (Lauche et al. 2017).

In traditional Chinese medicine, numerous other diseases—including cancer—are treated by a combination of qigong and conventional methods. Studies have shown an improvement in immune function (Wang et al. 2012) and positive effects on quality of life, mood and fatigue (Zeng et al. 2014) in cancer patients.

Comparing Tai Chi and Qigong, Tai Chi is more sport-oriented and has more effects in the direction of physical performance. Qigong is calmer and aims even more at relaxation (stress reduction). It is more of a cognitive intervention, whereas Medical Qigong is clearly disease-related.

Yoga

Yoga is over 5000 years old and has its origin in India. It consists of the main elements posture (Asana), breathing (Pranayama), meditation and "devotion" (Dhyana). Traditionally, six different styles of yoga (meditations, including transcendental meditations, mantra yoga) are practised in India. Various styles of yoga are also found in Western forms, but these are more body-oriented and usually closely related to asana (posture). They combine stretching and various postures with deep breathing and meditation. Hatha yoga (Hatha = sun/moon) is the most commonly practised style in the western world and consists mainly of relaxing exercises with physical strengthening.

There are excellent results from many studies (including Luu and Hall 2016) for western yoga: There is a reduction in blood pressure and heart rate, reduction in oxygen consumption, weight loss, strengthening of the legs, stress reduction, sleep improvement, reduction in anxiety, and memory improvement. Yoga is particularly suitable for the primary prevention of cardiovascular diseases (Cramer et al. 2014).

Thus, yoga shows excellent results in general prevention and secondary prevention. In pregnant women, yoga exercises lead to stress reduction, the reduction of hypertension and pain.

However, yoga is also successful in the treatment of pre-existing conditions and their rehabilitation: There is evidence for relevant positive effects on pain syndromes such as headache or arthritis pain (overview in Field 2011) and chronic, non-specific back pain (low back pain, Wieland et al. 2017). Therefore, yoga is recommended as an additional therapy in patients with low back pain. In addition, evidence is available for cardiovascular disease, autoimmune disease, cancer, metabolic syndrome and diabetes, fatigue, and hypertension. For major depression, yoga seems to be as effective as medication (Cramer et al. 2017).

The mechanisms of action of yoga are still largely unknown; it is assumed that it has a relaxing effect by controlling the sympathetic and parasympathetic nervous systems.

Yoga and Tai Chi also appear to have the potential to have a positive regulatory effect on the immune system and reduce inflammatory reactions. There are indications, but further studies are needed to ensure the evidence (Morgan et al. 2014).

Yoga exercises fit very well with the goals of forest therapy. However, an appropriate infrastructure with a solid floor and available mats are needed. Also, it should not be cold—according to the lighter clothing needed for most exercises.

Progressive Muscle Relaxation (PMR)

PMR is the most widespread relaxation method in Germany. The practitioner uses the fact that the muscles after a short tension easily pass into a perceptible state of relaxation. The practitioner should become a passive and careful observer of the relaxation process that occurs. PMR has been shown to affect pain, especially non-specific back pain. This led to the recommendation of PMR in the National German Health Care Guideline for Non-Specific Low Back Pain (2017). But the effectiveness of relaxation methods for chronic pain as a unimodal method is generally limited. However, it is very popular among pain patients in particular. When PMR is performed during forest therapy, it requires a quiet, dry place with a firm surface that is protected from noise and weather. And it must be warm so that the body does not cool down.

Autogenic Training

This relaxation method is mainly known in German-speaking countries. It is an autosuggestion procedure in which relaxation is induced by self-suggestion. Surprisingly, there are hardly any acceptable German or international studies on the effects (Ernst and Kanji 2000).

If autogenic training is to be practised during forest bathing or forest therapy, an appropriate infrastructure in the forest is necessary. Special attention must be paid to the fact that the practitioner lies completely still for a longer period (at least 20 min for the short form) and is thus at great risk of cooling down. In addition, to achieve the autosuggestion effect of total relaxation, absolute undisturbedness must prevail.

5.4.2   Climatotherapy, Climatotherapeutic Procedures

The "immersion in the atmosphere of the forest" is already by definition a part of climatotherapy. Shinrin-Yoku is very similar to what has long been practised in health resorts in the form of "air change" or "air baths"—scientifically: climatotherapy.

Climatotherapy belongs to the European and Japanese naturopathic healing methods and deals with the health-promoting effects of the climate on humans. Therefore, climate factors are well dosed to benefit from the individual climate factors for prevention, therapy and rehabilitation (Schuh 2004). The long-term successes of modern climatotherapy are largely documented and validated according to the criteria of "evidence-based medicine" (Schuh 2017). It is applied in the high mountain climate and the sea climate, but also the forest-dominated low mountain climate. In the forests, which are located around German spas and health resorts, climatotherapy is carried out in the form of fresh-air rest cures and climatic terrain treatments (see below). Today, climatotherapy is part of the outpatient treatment concept at the specialised health resorts with a healthy climate and it is prescribed by specialized physicians in health resort medicine or as a private preventive programme.

Thus, cures (formerly bathing cures, today outpatient preventive programmes) or rehabilitation programmes have been carried out in the wooded surroundings of German health resorts and spas for decades, titled "climatic therapy in the forest". Combined with other exercises, such as mindfulness to connect with nature, this is the perfect forest therapy!

Climatic Terrain Treatment
The actual goal of the so-called climatic terrain therapy or climatic terrain treatment is physical endurance training, which leads to increased performance. However, since forest therapy or forest bathing is designed to be rather quiet, the training must also be reduced. Thus a terrain treatment "light" is carried out with low intensities resp. with low walking speed. However, if—in the sense of the "climatic terrain treatment"—the relaxed walking in the shady forest is carried out with the inclusion of the forest climate factor" cool air", then excellent effects are to be expected. Even without physical exertion, an increase in physical performance is achieved (Schuh 2004). The increased endurance capacity is caused by the slight cooling of the skin during a relaxed hike. The cooling is regulated via clothing. This "cool body shell" affects circulation and muscle metabolism and increases the health-promoting effects of the walk. It also has an exercise effect on the thermoregulatory system (see

Sect. 3.4), which leads to the physical change known as hardening (see Sect. 5.4.3).

Fresh-Air Rest Cure

The even more important climate exposure procedure for forest therapy is the fresh-air rest cure. It was formerly used to treat pulmonary tuberculosis. The aim was the "training en repos" ("training while resting"), which should result in general strengthening. Today, the fresh-air rest cure is mainly used for prevention, but also strengthening, e.g. convalescents, weakened or old people or also people with walking difficulties.

The physical basis of the fresh-air rest cure is resting, combined with slightly reduced skin temperature, which leads to significant physical relaxation. Although undertaken without simultaneous physical activity, the fresh-air rest cure also leads to a slight increase in physical performance (Schuh 2004). As the term "training en repos" already suggests, this general strengthening results from the physical relaxation and subsequent regeneration that occurs during serial resting in cool air.

The conditions in the forest offer excellent opportunities for this, either by just sitting or lying down quietly in the forest or during body-mind exercises (see Sect. 5.4.1), during which you move only a little or hardly at all. In this case, the reduced skin temperature leads to simultaneous physical strengthening. However, especially at rest, strict attention must be paid to ensure that the body does not cool down.

5.4.3   Kneipp Therapy

Kneipp therapy, like climatotherapy, belongs to the traditional European healing methods. It is composed of the 5 pillars of Kneipp therapy: water (hydrotherapy), nutrition (dietetics), medicinal herbs (phytotherapy), movement (exercise therapy) and body-mind-spiritual medicine (German "Ordnungstherapie").

Kneipp therapy was developed in the nineteenth century by Sebastian Kneipp (1821–1897), a catholic pastor in Bad Wörishofen. He developed an individual therapy system as a regulation therapy with the focus of the improvement of the body's own healing process, mainly by cold water applications. He is said to have cured himself of pulmonary tuberculosis with it.

Today, Kneipp therapy is carried out as part of cures in special health resort facilities, as an accompaniment to other cure regimes, but also at home.

Hydrotherapy

The basis of hydrotherapy is that the element water, as a mediator of natural life stimuli, increases performance, stimulates the immune system and improves body awareness. Water treatments have a preventive and therapeutic harmonizing effect on the nervous and hormonal system as well as on the psyche. The applications are extremely differentiated—over 100 are known. They are described in Brüggemann and Uehleke (1997), among others.

Hydrotherapeutic elements, such as treading water in a stream or dew treading in a clearing, are an ideal enrichment of forest therapy during the summer months. For treading water, however, there should be a paved entrance to the stream and, if necessary, a handrail.

Exercise Therapy

It was first introduced in Kneipp therapy as a preparatory action and as rewarming after cold applications. The exercises should be dynamic and consist of walking, running, swimming, cycling, etc. The movement should be enjoyable, fit into the lifestyle and be able to be continued at home (Brüggemann and Uehleke 1997).

During forest therapy, there are excellent opportunities to exercise repeatedly in the form of light walks, preferably as a climatic terrain treatment (see Sect. 5.4.2). Especially in the transitional seasons and in winter, movement therapy/exercises are indispensable to protect the participants from cooling down.

Body-Mind-Spiritual Medicine ("Ordnungstherapie")

Pastor Kneipp himself understood this kind of regulative therapy of inner balance as "bringing order to the soul" and set the goal: "Ordnungstherapie should take care that the soul remains or becomes whole". Then as now, this body-mind-spiritual medicine should teach people to live in harmony with themselves and the environment, to understand life crises as opportunities for development and to make course corrections, and to see ageing as the counted time that should be used: Pause, see and do what is essential, considering the fascination of slowness. Today's goal of this regulative therapy is the restoration of a natural individual life order, i.e. building a healthy lifestyle. Modern "Ordnungstherapie" thus primarily aims at behavioural changes, i.e. the modification of the previous lifestyle by becoming aware of interrelationships. This includes emotional and interactive components such as the teaching of social, emotional and communicative skills, but also a somatic component in the form of training physiological parameters through exercise, relaxation, nutrition and breathing, among others. Living according to chronobiological findings ("chronohygiene") and sleep management is also important.

The contents of the Kneipp body-mind-spiritual therapy corresponds to the goals that are to be conveyed during the forest therapy with body-mind procedures and mindfulness practise used.

Phytotherapy and Nutritional Therapy

Pastor Kneipp also introduced phytotherapy. Even today, mildly acting herbs/plants, their parts or extracts are still used for internal and external medical applications and are used as remedies, for prevention, or as care products. As a supplement to forest therapy, phytotherapeutics can be used for stress reduction and calming as well as for good sleep.

Nutritional therapy is another pillar of Kneipp therapy. Here it is about dietetics according to modern nutritional physiology, about the order of meals with a cultivated, rhythmic intake as well as about the sensual pleasure of eating.

Effects

The effectiveness of Kneipp therapy has been confirmed in numerous studies (e.g. Uehleke et al. 2008). Especially for patients with high blood pressure (Jacob and Volger 2009) and other cardiovascular diseases (Leuchtgens et al. 1999) significant improvements are known. Older people, who often suffer from several diseases, also benefit excellently from Kneipp therapy (Weigl et al. 2008). However, Kneipp therapy is particularly successful in general prevention and the sense of hardening (Goedsche et al. 2007), including chronic obstructive bronchitis. Numerous results are available in this regard.

In Shinrin-Yoku, Kneipp therapy can be an excellent supporting component. For example, careful arm or foot baths in a stream flowing through the forest support or train the thermoregulatory system (see Sect. 3.4). The thoughts of "Ordnungstherapie" should be consolidated in combination with body-mind procedures or mindfulness training. Light exercise therapy in the form of the climatic terrain treatment (see above) or light walks, healthy nutrition or teas made from forest herbs further promote the effects of Shinrin-Yoku.

5.5   Rights of Using a Forest Based on German Regulations

The German federal forest act does not yet contain any specific provisions for the use of the forest as a cure or healing forest as well as forest therapy purposes (Bundesministerium der Justiz und für Verbraucherschutz 2021). The only exception is the state Mecklenburg-Western Pomerania, which, in addition to a useful, protective and recreational function, has also anchored the health function in their state forest law (Section 22 of the State Forest Act M-V) since 2011. Otherwise, the responsible local (forestry) authority examines on a case-by-case basis whether a site can be approved. The prerequisite is always that the useful, protective and recreational functions of the forest are not impaired by forest bathing.

Complex questions arise about the framework conditions. This concerns the commercial practice of forest therapy programmes. For the designation and implementation of cure and healing forests, specific aspects are added. For the first time, Volz et al. (2018) have summarised this very complex topic for the different actors in Germany as an orientation. However, this is merely an overview of the most important and known framework conditions, does not claim completeness, and excludes liability claims against the authors.

5.5.1   General Framework Conditions Under German Forest Law for the Professional Practice of Forest Therapy

In principle, for any commercial use of the forest (forest bathing, forest therapy, Shinrin-Yoku) the legal requirements have to be observed and implemented.

In connection with forest therapy intervention, completely new risks and obligations may arise for the provider, but also for the forest owner:

Property Law Aspect: The Right of Use
The implementation of forest therapy programmes (e.g. by health resorts, tourist offices, hotels or in the form of self-employment, e.g. as a forest health trainer or forest therapist) constitutes a commercial use that is not covered by the right of access under Section 14 of the German Federal Forest Act and is therefore only permissible with the consent of the forest owners concerned. Anyone wishing to offer forest therapy programmes, but who is not the owner of a forest himself, is dependent on acquiring or leasing the forest area required

for the implementation of forest therapy programmes or acquiring the necessary rights of use from the landowner by contract (e.g. using so-called permission contracts).

Therefore, it is recommended for a commercial forest therapy project to secure it through corresponding long-term permission contracts with the respective forest owners, to notify the responsible (forestry) authorities at an early stage and to coordinate the plans with them.

Lease and Permission Agreements

In the case of a lease agreement, the lessee takes over the entire use of the forest land (including forest management, which can be transferred to a forestry service provider, for example).

In the case of a permit contract, only the respective special use is regulated, while forest management remains with the forest owner. Permit agreements can be freely formulated; they should regulate the exact use as well as the rights and obligations of the user and owner in a binding manner. As a rule, this includes stipulating exactly what use of the forest is envisaged and what the forest owner has to do, to tolerate or refrain from doing (hunting, type and extent of forest management, traffic safety).

Nature Conservation and Species Protection Requirements

In addition to property and trespassing rights, nature conservation and species protection regulations also have generally valid aspects that limit the granting of permits:

Forest areas may be subject to different *protection statuses* (e.g. nature conservation area, nature park, flora-fauna habitat or bird sanctuary). It is therefore necessary to clarify in advance whether a protection category applies. This applies not only to protected areas under nature conservation law, but also, for example, to protected areas under forest law (e.g. protective forest, recreational forest, ban forest, natural forest reserves) or underwater protection law. Water protection areas are subject to special requirements, as they serve to protect surface and underground water resources from adverse impacts (Section 51 (1) of the Federal Water Act).

Certain native animal and plant species are protected under the German *Nature and Species Protection Act.* According to § 44 paragraph, 1 no. 2 of the Federal Nature Conservation Act, for example, it is prohibited to significantly disturb wild animals of strictly protected species and European bird species during the breeding, rearing, moulting, hibernation and migration periods. In such cases, the statutory protection of nature and species takes precedence over the interest of use. For example, the nature conservation authority may order that certain forest areas (e.g. eyrie protection zone) may not be entered at certain times of the year.

Nature conservation and species protection regulations can thus decisively determine under which conditions and to what extent a forest therapy project can be implemented on a specific forest area. Nature conservation and species protection concerns should therefore be clarified with the local nature conservation authorities at an early stage. On this basis, a concept can be developed that takes account of nature conservation concerns by leaving out sensitive areas, steering critical activities in a nature-compatible direction and flanking the forest therapy project, for example, with a "sanitation and waste concept".

Right of Access to the Forest
In principle, the forest in Germany may be entered without restriction for recreation according to § 14 of the German Federal Forest Act (Bundesministerium der Justiz und für Verbraucherschutz 2021). This also applies to a private forest. This general right of access also applies outside of the paths and without limitation of time and must be accepted by the forest owner and other authorised users (e.g. hunters or operators of forest therapy services). It can therefore only be restricted for important reasons specifically described in the forest laws of the Federal Government or the respective states (forest protection, forest or hunting management, protection of forest visitors, avoidance of considerable damage; German Federal Forest Act § 14 paragraph 2).

However, providers of forest therapy programmes should take into account in their planning that entering the forest can often be affected by forest closures that cannot be planned, e.g. in the event of acute forest fire danger, storms, danger due to snow breakage or infestation by pests (oak processionary moth). In addition, forest visits should not take place at dusk, at night or dawn out of consideration for other interest groups, animals and also for personal protection (see also Chap. 6).

Road Safety Obligation
As a general rule, forest visitors enter the forest for recreational purposes at their own risk (§ 14 paragraph 1, German Federal Forest Act) (Bundesministerium der Justiz und für Verbraucherschutz 2021). Thus, in the forest and on the corresponding paths, there is no duty to ensure safety and no liability on the part of the forest owner for hazards typical of the forest and special hazards resulting from nature.

The commercial use of the forest is no longer covered by the general exemption of the Federal Forest Act, from the duty of road safety and liability. Thus, the provider of forest therapy interventions, and possibly also the forest owner who allows the use, have a special responsibility for the road safety of the forests or forest sections used. Providers of forest therapy services and forest owners involved are therefore well advised to address the issue of road safety to counter typical forest hazards through appropriate safety measures.

5.5.2 Special Legal Requirements for Cure or Healing Forest in Germany

Forestry Regulations

So far, only in the German State Mecklenburg-Western Pomerania is it possible to designate and declare cure and healing forests as a separate legal category through a legal ordinance (Section 22 of the State Forest Act of Mecklenburg-Western Pomerania). Furthermore, the German federal forest act does not (so far) contain any specific provisions for the use of the forest as a cure or healing forest (Bundesministerium der Justiz und für Verbraucherschutz 2021). Nevertheless, the use of the forest as a therapeutic refuge appears to be possible and permissible in principle, as long as—as described above—other uses, protection and recreational functions of the forest are not impaired. For the approval of cure and healing forests, the responsible local (forestry) authority must therefore be consulted in each case.

In order to enable and facilitate this examination, it is recommended that those interested in developing cure and healing forests, in addition to clarifying the general prerequisites (see above), describe the intended project as concretely as possible so that all relevant aspects can be included. This includes knowledge about the owner, the suitability, location and size of the forest area(s), group size, target groups (prevention or special indications), a description of the specific intervention and necessary infrastructure measures and their approvability as well as a possible visitor guidance concept (see Sect. 5.2).

Possible Interventions in the Forest

In principle, it is advisable to be as cautious as possible with regard to structural constructions in the forest and to coordinate them with all parties concerned at an early stage. However, depending on the type and size of the planned cure or healing forest and the target group, a certain structural infrastructure within the forest may be indispensable (e.g. rescue or shelter huts, sanitary facilities). Facilities and infrastructure in the vicinity of the forest could also be used. This requires appropriate agreements or user contracts. It should also be borne in mind that, in addition to the initial investment, any infrastructure that is built will also require a high level of care, maintenance and upkeep over the long term, and may also entail special obligations to ensure road safety.

The construction of structural facilities in the forest can result in a considerable and, above all, permanent impairment of the natural balance. This applies in principle to the entire forest area, even outside protected areas. According to § 13 ff. Federal Nature Conservation Act, interventions in the natural balance must be avoided as a matter of principle and as a matter of priority; significant impairments that cannot be avoided must be compensated employing compensatory or replacement measures.

Therefore, when planning cure and healing forests, care should be taken from the outset to use the naturally existing conditions of the respective forest area and to avoid construction measures or the erection of artificial structures as far as possible.

As cure and healing forests, the corresponding forest areas may be frequented much more by visitors. From the point of view of nature conservation and species protection, this generally means a possible disturbance of the forest's fauna as well as an increased burden on the flora, e.g. through trampling damage, picking, tearing and soil compaction. In addition, the use of the forest for therapeutic purposes could also lead to increased inputs of waste and of non-forest pathogens, nitrogen and drug residues (e.g. by defecating in the forest).

Road Safety Obligation

The forest is a natural area with typical forest hazards. Not only healthy visitors stay in a cure or healing forest, but also elderly seniors or patients who may be restricted in their ability to move as well as in their ability to see and hear due to age and/or illness. As already described, the duty of care and liability are not covered by the German Federal Forest Act (Bundesministerium der Justiz und für Verbraucherschutz 2021). As a result, the operators of cure and healing forests are faced with special tasks (security issues and liability aspects) to be able to carry out forest therapy programmes.

References[1]

3sat (2019) Therapie unter Tannen. Die geheimnisvolle Kraft der Bäume. Wissenschaftdoku. http://www.3sat.de/mediathek/?mode=play&obj=66178. Accessed 29 Mar 2019

Allmer H (1996) Erholung und Gesundheit: Grundlagen, Ergebnisse und Maßnahmen. Hogrefe, Göttingen

Bauer N, Roe J, Martens D (2016) Der Einfluss von physischer Umwelt auf den Menschen: Erholung, Wohlbefinden, Gesundheit und Lebensqualität. Umweltpsychologie 20:3–14

Beckmann J, Fröhlich SM (2009) Erholung und Stressmanagment. In: Wippert P, Beckmann J (Eds) Stress- und Schmerzursachen verstehen. http://www.beck-shop.de/fachbuch/leseprobe/9783131440112_Excerpt_003.pdf.   Accessed 29 Mar 2019

Braun A (2000) Die Wahrnehmung von Wald und Natur. Forschung Soziologie 58. Springer, Heidelberg

Brüggemann W, Uehleke B (1997) Kneipp Vademecum pro Medico: Hydrotherapie, Phytotherapie, Bewegungstherapie, Ernährung, Ordnungstherapie. Sebastian Kneipp Gesundheitsmittel, Bad Wörishofen

Bundesministerium der Justiz und für Verbraucherschutz (2021) Bundeswaldgesetz. http://www.gesetze-im-internet.de/bwaldg/BJNR010370975.html.   Accessed 22 Aug 2021

Chodzko-Zajko WJ, Proctor DN, Fiatarone Singh MA, Minson CT, Nigg CR, Salem GJ, Skinner JS (2009) American College of Sports Medicine position stand. Exercise and physical activity for older adults. Med Sci Sports Exerc 41:1510–1530

Cramer H, Lauche R, Haller H, Steckhan N, Michalsen A, Dobos G (2014) Effects of yoga on cardiovascular disease risk factors: a systematic review and meta-analysis. Int J Cardiol 173(2):170–183

Cramer H, Lauche R, Klose P, Lange S, Langhorst J, Dobos GJ (2017) Yoga for improving health-related quality of life, mental health and cancer-related symptoms in women diagnosed with breast cancer. Cochrane Database Syst Rev 1:CD010802

Ernst E, Kanji N (2000) Autogenic training for stress and anxiety: a systematic review. Complement Ther Med 8:106–110

Esch T (2014) Die neuronale Basis von Meditation und Achtsamkeit. Sucht 60:21–28

Field T (2011) Yoga clinical research review. Complement Ther Clin Pract 17:1–8

Franzkowiak P (2018) Prävention und Krankheitsprävention. BZgA Leitbegriffe der Gesundheitsförderung.   https://www.leitbegriffe.bzga.de/systematisches-verzeichnis/allgemeine-grundbegriffe/praevention-und-krankheitspraevention/. Accessed 15 Mar 2019

---

[1] For the legal texts, the respective current publications on the internet apply.

Goedsche K, Förster M, Kroegel C, Uhlemann C (2007) Repeated cold water stimulations (hydrotherapy according to Kneipp) in patients with COPD. Forsch Komplementmed 14:158–166

Goyal M, Singh S, Sibinga EM, Gould NF, Rowland-Seymour A, Sharma R, Berger Z, Sleicher D, Maron DD, Shihab HM, Ranasinghe PD, Linn S, Saha S, Bass EB, Haythornthwaite JA (2015) Meditation programs for psychological stress and well-being: a systematic review and meta-analysis. JAMA Intern Med 174:357–368

Guan H, Wei H, He X, Ren Z, An B (2017) The tree-species-specific effect of forest bathing on perceived anxiety alleviation of young-adults in urban forests. Ann For Res 60:327–341

Hofmann M, Gerstenberg T, Gillner S (2017) Predicting tree preferences from visible tree characteristics. Eur J For Res 136:421–432

Huang ZG, Feng YH, Li YH, Lv CS (2017) Systematic review and meta-analysis: Tai Chi for preventing falls in older adults. BMJ Open 7:e013661

Hui SS, Woo J, Kwok T (2009) Evaluation of energy expenditure and cardiovascular health effects from Tai Chi and walking exercise. Hong Kong Med J 15(Suppl 2):4–7

Jacob EM, Volger E (2009) Blutdrucksenkung durch Hydrotherapie. Z Phys Med Rehabil Kurortmed 19:162–168

Kaiser AA (2016) Entwicklung und Evaluation selbstinstruktiver Körper-Achtsamkeitsprogramme zur Gesundheitsförderung und Erholung am Arbeitsplatz. Dissertation, Pädagogischen Hochschule Karlsruhe

Khoury B, Sharma M, Rush SE, Fournier C (2015) Mindfulness-based stress reduction for healthy individuals: a meta-analysis. J Psychosom Res 78:519–528

Kleinhückelkotten S, Neitzke HP (2010) Naturbewusstsein 2009. Abschlussbericht. ECOLOG-Institut für sozial-ökologische Forschung, Berlin/Bonn

Lan C, Chen SY, Lai JS (2008) The exercise intensity of Tai Chi Chuan. Med Sport Sci 52:12–19

Lauche R, Peng W, Ferguson C, Cramer H, Frawley J, Adams J, Sibbritt D (2017) Efficacy of Tai Chi and qigong for the prevention of stroke and stroke risk factors: a systematic review with meta-analysis. Medicine (Baltimore) 96:e8517

Leuchtgens H, Albus T, Uhlemann C, Volger E, Pelka RB, Resch KL (1999) Auswirkungen der Kneipp-Kur, einer standardisierten Komplextherapie, auf Schmerz, Lebensqualität und Medikamentenverbrauch: Kohortenstudie mit 1-Jahres-follow-up. Forsch Komplementmed 6:206–211

Liu T, Chan AW, Liu YH, Taylor-Piliae RE (2018) Effects of Tai Chi-based cardiac rehabilitation on aerobic endurance, psychosocial well-being, and cardiovascular risk reduction among patients with coronary heart disease: a systematic review and meta-analysis. Eur J Cardiovasc Nurs 17:368–383

Lupp G, Förster B, Kantelberg V, Weber G, Pauleit S (2017) Stadtwald 2050. Endbericht. Lehrstuhl für Strategie und Management der Landschaftsentwicklung, Wissenschaftszentrum Weihenstephan, Technische Universität München

Luu K, Hall PA (2016) Hatha yoga and executive function: a systematic review. J Altern Complement Med 22:125–133

Morgan N, Irwin MR, Chung M, Wang C (2014) The effects of mind-body therapies on the immune system: meta-analysis. PLoS One 9:e100903

Nationale Versorgungs-Leitlinie (2017) Kreuzschmerz. AWMF-Register: nvl/007. www.leitlinien.de/mdb/downloads/nvl/kreuzschmerz/kreuzschmerz-2aufl-vers1-lang.pdf. Accessed 29 Mar 2019

Ng BH, Tsang HW (2009) Psychophysiological outcomes of health qigong for chronic conditions: a systematic review. Psychophysiology 46:257–269

Schuh A (2004) Klima- und Thalassotherapie: Grundlagen und Praxis. Hippokrates, Stuttgart

Schuh A (2017) Klimatherapie Grundlagen und Praxis. In: Kraft K, Stange R (eds) Kursbuch Naturheilverfahren für die ärztliche Weiterbildung. Elsevier, Munich

Schuh A, Immich G (2013) Kriterienkatalog für Kur- Heilwälder. Im Auftrag des Bäderverbandes von Mecklenburg-Vorpommern. Ludwig-Maximilians-Universität, München

Takayama N, Fujiwara A, Saito H, Horiuchi M (2017) Management effectiveness of a secondary coniferous forest for landscacpe appreciation and psychological restoration. Int J Environ Res Public Health 14:800

Uehleke B, Wöhling H, Stange R (2008) A prospective "study by correspondence" on the effects of Kneipp hydrotherapy in patients with complaints due to polyneuropathy. Schweizer Z Ganzheitsmed 20:287–291

Volz HA, Immich G, Schuh A (2018) Kur-/Heiwälder: eine Chance für Waldeigentümer. Allg Forstzeitschrift Waldwirtschaft Umweltvorsorge 16:10–13

Wang CW, Ng SM, Ho RT, Ziea ET, Wong VC, Chan CL (2012) The effect of qigong exercise on immunity and infections: a systematic review of controlled trials. Am J Chin Med 40:1143–1156

Weigl M, Ewert T, Kleinschmidt J, Stucki G (2008) Ambulante Medizinische Kuren in bayerischen Heilbädern: Eine multizentrische, prospektive Kohortenstudie mit 3-monatigem Follow-up. Z Phys Med Rehabil Kurortmed 18:127–135

Weitmann V, Korny D (2014) Die Erholungseignung des Auwaldes – Untersuchung der Besucher-Aktivitäten und Bewertung von unterschiedlichen Waldbildern in den Isar-Auwäldern nördlich von München. Projektarbeit am Lehrstuhl für Strategie und Management der Landschaftsentwicklung, Technische Universität München

Wieland LS, Skoetz N, Pilkington K, Vempati R, D'Adamo CR, Berman BM (2017) Yoga treatment for chronic non-specific low back pain. Cochrane Database Syst Rev 1:CD010671

Yeh GY, Mietus JE, Peng CK, Phillips RS, Davis RB, Wayne PM, Goldberger AL, Thomas RJ (2008) Enhancement of sleep stability with Tai Chi exercise in chronic heart failure: preliminary findings using an ECG-based spectrogram method. Sleep Med 9:527–536

Zeng Y, Luo T, Xie H, Huang M, Cheng AS (2014) Health benefits of qigong or Tai Chi for cancer patients: a systematic review and meta-analysis. Complement Ther Med 22:173–186

Zou L, Sasaki JE, Wei GX, Huang T, Yeung AS, Neto OB, Chen KW, Hui SS (2018) Effects of mind-body exercises (Tai Chi/Yoga) on heart rate variability parameters and perceived stress: a systematic review with meta-analysis of randomized controlled trials. J Clin Med 31:11

6

Risks and Potential Dangers in the Forest

Summary

The forest is used for recreational and health purposes, but it is not completely safe. It is therefore important to familiarise oneself with possible dangers, e.g. from ticks or weather events or forces of nature, in advance of a visit to the forest and to adapt one's behaviour accordingly. This also includes taking appropriate protective precautions (clothing, tick spray, etc.) and, if necessary, postponing the visit to the forest or leaving the forest immediately.

The absence of danger during the stay in the forest must be ensured. Only those who feel safe can relax and recover. If safety is ensured, then being alone in the forest is beneficial for mental recuperation, especially in the case of psychological exhaustion, and for relaxation.

But women often do not like to go into the forest alone. Childhood experiences probably also play a certain role in whether one goes into the forest and how one feels about it (Staats and Hartig 2004). Here, the accompaniment of a known person can increase the feeling of security.

6.1 Risk Factors

Storms, thunderstorms, and intense snowfall pose a significant potential hazard. Anyone who spends time outdoors for work or leisure should be aware of the great danger posed by lightning strikes in the forest during thunderstorms.

© Springer-Verlag GmbH Germany, part of Springer Nature 2022
A. Schuh, G. Immich, *Forest Therapy - The Potential of the Forest for Your Health*,
https://doi.org/10.1007/978-3-662-64280-1_6

Although people often believe that they are protected under the trees, there is great danger in the forest and especially at the forest edge! If lightning strikes a tree, it conducts the energy along the trunk, from which it "jumps" to a person located under the tree. However, the energy of the lightning can also be conducted into the roots and from there into the surrounding area and endanger people standing there (Deutscher Wetterdienst 2017).

In the event of a storm, the forest should also be left as quickly as possible or not entered at all! Even with only moderate wind, cones or dead branches can break off. They can twist in the air due to gravity, then fall vertically like an arrow and cause serious injury or even fatal injury to the forest visitor. Falling branches thus represent an often underestimated source of danger. In the event of a storm, forest visitors may also be in danger of death if a tree suddenly falls (windthrow), even if the tree breaks off in the trunk area (wind breakage).

Snow load on the trees, under which they can collapse or fall over and branches break off, are also very dangerous. Forest fire risk is often underestimated. Mixed hardwood stands on moist or fresh valley sites are therefore less at risk than pure coniferous stands. The prohibition of open fires and smoking in the forest is regulated differently depending on the national German federal state, and is valid either all year round or from March 1, to October 31 (ban of smoking or any open fire in the forest). But even in the dry winters open fire in the forest is "fire danger". This has been shown by large winter forest fires, e.g. in the Bavarian Alps, caused by a campfire in a mountain forest.

Cautious behaviour in the forest is essential. This includes, among other things, not climbing on outdoor seats and wooden poles.

It is also possible that various plants hurt the forest visitor: Giant hogweed, an umbellifer, grows more than three meters tall in a few weeks, and the leaves reach a length of 1 m or more. The dangerous substance is the fucomarines present in the plant sap, which have a phototoxic effect mainly on the skin in combination with sunlight. The skin symptoms resemble severe burns with strong reddening and blistering and must be treated medically. Even touching the skin in daylight can cause painful wheals and blisters in sensitive people. Children are particularly at risk because the hollow plant stems and the giant leaves tempt them to play and hide.

But hemlock, datura, buttercups, belladonna, red and blue monkshood, daphne, crocus, yew, miracle tree, poison ivy and laburnum, among others, are also toxic to varying degrees (Pahlow 2006).

In addition to valuable mushrooms, fruits and plants, there are also a lot of harmful or poisonous ones in the forest. Mushrooms, berries and leaves should only be collected or eaten if you have precise knowledge of the plant.

Mosquitoes are present in the forest. The high humidity increases the activity of mosquitoes and their ability to transmit diseases. But other animal sources of danger are also possible. These include aggressive wild boars or snakes such as the adder. There may also be poisonous spiders or hornets in the forest. The oak or pine processionary moth poses a mostly local threat. On its body surface, there are so-called stinging hairs with barbs, which cause local skin rashes with itching and burning at the point of contact. Irritation of the mouth and nasal mucous membranes may also occur due to inhalation of the hairs, resulting in bronchitis, painful coughing and even asthma. The hairs can easily be carried up to several hundred meters by the wind and are still effective even after months. Due to climate change, the caterpillars of both moths are expected to continue to spread. All animals that just have young can attack to defend themselves.

Within the framework of more or less serious offers of forest bathing, recommendations are increasingly being made to go into the forest at night. The nocturnal environment and darkness in the forest are to be used for relaxation or self-discovery, for example. However, this is not without danger, because in addition to nocturnal animals, there have recently been many hunters in the forests.

In the context of increased engagement with nature, it currently seems to be "in" to acquire a hunting license (2017/18: 384,429 hunting license holders and per hunter 214 inhabitants; Deutscher Jagdverband 2018). Thus, although more and more people are going hunting, they are not experienced and can thus pose a danger to "forest bathers", especially at dusk and at night, but also in the early morning hours.

6.2 Diseases

In rare cases, spending time in the forest can also be detrimental to health or even cause illness. Biogenic, potentially harmful air components can be present in the forest, as plants and trees emit larger and smaller biogenic particles. These are dust formed from plant residues such as leaves, but above all plant seeds and pollen, which can be transported over long distances in the air.

Since conifer pollens are also allergenic, allergy sufferers are also affected by flying pollen during the flowering period of their allergen-relevant trees in the forest. This is just not generally known because conifer pollens are very large and therefore heavy and quickly sinks to the ground in the forest. Unlike other flower or grass pollen, the conifer pollens are not transported far away. In heavy rain/wind or thunderstorms, the pollens are broken up and the proteins fly around. This massively increases allergenicity (D'Amato et al. 2015). Therefore, conifer pollen allergy sufferers should not go into the forest during the seasonal pollen season and also not during or after heavy rain.

Since the entire nature, especially the forest floor and the plants, are alive with microorganisms, every time they are stirred up, microorganisms can naturally enter the air. They are found as isolated individual particles in the air. Frequently, these are fungus-spores. Fungi or moulds grow at high humidity on almost all organic substrates. From its air-mycelium, the spores can be released already with small air movements. Because they are relatively resistant, they remain viable longer than other germs. Mould allergy sufferers can thus experience a worsening of symptoms in the forest, especially during autumn leaves.

Other microorganisms, especially bacteria and yeasts, adhere to solid particles such as soil particles, plant parts, or faeces. In addition, they can be released in the form of droplets by humans and animals or by wind movements from water containing germs. Birds are also carriers of microorganisms and parasites.

Eating wild strawberries or raspberries, for example, can cause a rather rare infection with the eggs of the fox tapeworm. Sick animals such as rabid foxes can attack you and transmit diseases.

Diseases and infections transmitted naturally between animals and humans (zoonoses) will increase due to globalisation and climate change. To date, approximately 200 zoonoses are known. Appropriate information about preventive measures (clothing, protective means, behaviour, careful handling of animals and natural fruits) is therefore important to minimise the risk!

This also applies in particular to protection against ticks, which transmit the most important forest-related diseases worldwide: Lyme disease and early summer meningoencephalitis. Ticks, which are stripped by humans from hedges, bushes or grass, are already active from air temperatures of 6 °C. In recent decades, ticks have appeared in higher numbers in the Czech Republic and even in higher altitude areas of Sweden. Due to climate change, air temperatures will continue to increase and summers are expected to become longer and warmer. Therefore, ticks can penetrate further north and thus spread further and further in the northern hemisphere. In addition, the survival rate of the tick is increased by milder winters and a longer vegetation period.

Lyme disease is the most common infectious disease transmitted by ticks (common wood tick) in Central Europe. It is widespread in the northern hemisphere (North America, Europe, and Asia). Today, it can already be assumed that there is a risk of infection in all parts of Germany. Lyme disease is caused by bacteria (Borrelia burgdorferi). About 17% of ticks in Germany are carriers of the pathogen. Hosts are especially rodents, some bird species as well as wild animals—the ticks then transmit the infection from the host to humans. The number of Lyme disease cases caused by tick bites in Bavaria, for example, increased by 40% in 2018 compared to the previous year. Extrapolating this to case numbers for Germany, this means 80,000–120,000 new Lyme disease cases per year (Deutscher Bundestag 2017). Lyme disease shows a pronounced seasonality due to the temperature-dependent activity of ticks from April onwards, peaking in August. With climate change, the tick-active period will expand.

The second disease that can be transmitted by a tick bite is spring-summer meningoencephalitis (or tick-born encephalitis TBE). Here, however, the infestation of ticks with the TBE virus has so far been low in Germany, and 1–2 cases/100,000 people occur, depending on the climate and recreational behaviour (Robert Koch Institute 2019). So far, the most frequent TBE cases are still recorded in Bavaria and Baden-Württemberg; individual cases also occur in other German federal states. Currently, approximately 600 cases of TBE are reported throughout Germany, of which 30% show signs of illness and 10% take a severe course (impfen-info.de 2019). The Robert Koch Institute publishes an annual map of the current TBE risk areas in Germany.

The forest as a living and recreational space can therefore be dangerous. In addition to dangerous or sick animals or animals carrying disease, the forest also contains a wide variety of fungi, fruits, and berries which, if not known, can cause moderate to lethal damage to health. To be able to avoid all risk factors and dangers in the forest preventively or to counteract them appropriately, it is, therefore, necessary to have well-trained specialists who inform and protect people during forest therapy.

References

D'Amato G, Holgate ST, Pawankar R, Ledford DK, Cecchi L, Al-Ahmad M, Al-Enezi F, Al-Muhsen S, Ansotegui I, Baena-Cagnani CE, Baker DJ, Bayram H, Bergmann KC, Boulet LP, Buters JT, D'Amato M, Dorsano S, Douwes J, Finlay SE, Garrasi D, Gómez M, Haahtela T, Halwani R, Hassani Y, Mahboub B, Marks G, Michelozzi P, Montagni M, Nunes C, Oh JJ, Popov TA, Portnoy J, Ridolo E, Rosário N, Rottem M, Sánchez-Borges M, Sibanda E, Sienra-Monge JJ, Vitale C, Annesi-Maesano I (2015) Meteorological conditions, climate change, new emerging factors, and asthma and related allergic disorders. A statement of the World Allergy Organization. World Allergy Organ J 8:5

Deutscher Bundestag (2017) Sachstand zur Lyme-Borreliose. https://www.bundestag.de/resource/blob/510388/baa593c34d8a69b231021ab2db95a208/wd-9-012-17-pdf-data.pdf. Accessed 22 Jan 2019

Deutscher Jagdverband (2018) Zahl der Jagdscheininhaber. https://www.jagdverband.de/content/jagdscheininhaber-deutschland. Accessed 20 Feb 2018

Deutscher Wetterdienst (2017) Gewitter, Blitze und persönliche Verhaltensregeln. https://www.dwd.de/DE/wetter/thema_des_tages/2017/5/11.html.   Accessed 31 Mar 2019

Impf-Info.de (2019) Impfempfehlungen für Erwachsene für FSME. www.impfen-info.de/impfempfehlungen/fuer-erwachsene/fsme-fruehsommer-meningoenzephalitis/. Accessed 31 Mar 2019

Pahlow M (2006) Das große Buch der Heilpflanzen. Gräfe & Unzer, Munich

Robert Koch-Institut (2019) FSME Früh-Sommer-Meningoenzephalitis. https://www.rki.de/DE/Content/infAZ/F/FSME/FSME-node. Accessed 23 Feb 2019

Staats H, Hartig T (2004) Alone or with a friend: a social context for psychological restoration and environmental preferences. J Environ Psychol 24:199–211

7

Conclusion and Outlook

Summary

Forest therapy is becoming more and more important in Germany, because it picks up on an ancient German theme again. The forest has always played an elementary role in the German history: People have lived in forests, it gave protection and provided them with food and wood for fire and building, and today it represents a major economic factor. Forest visits bring people "back to nature" (Rousseau 1722–1778) and offer opportunities for balance and recharging in our modern times. A forest is a place of retreat from the hectic life, one can come to rest, "let the soul dangle" and at the same time draw new strength. Visits to the forest allow a new approach to nature, even in a technological world. Moreover, a stay in the forest is possible without extensive preparations, it does not cause any major costs for the "forest bathers", and one does not need any special sports clothing or equipment.

Forest therapy will become more and more established in Germany and worldwide, a massive trend is already emerging.

A lot is already known and scientifically supported about the preventive benefits of forest therapy on emotional, psychological and physical risk factors. It can be considered that forest therapy has a calming and relaxing effect and reduces stress. This is of great importance because of our busy and demanding modern life and justifies the increasing interest in forest therapy, both in the public and in professional circles.

© Springer-Verlag GmbH Germany, part of Springer Nature 2022
A. Schuh, G. Immich, *Forest Therapy - The Potential of the Forest for Your Health*,
https://doi.org/10.1007/978-3-662-64280-1_7

Soon, however, the aim must be to expand the range of applications of forest therapy and to investigate whether forest therapy also has demonstrable short- or long-term effects on various existing illnesses. The focus here is on manifest mental illnesses such as depression. On the physical side, there are nowadays increasing diseases of the respiratory tract, in the cardiovascular system, or the metabolic area. These diseases are promoted by environmental pollution, but also lifestyle. Forest therapy with the relieving elements of the forest climate and the activities carried out in it (including relaxation, mindfulness practice, light exercise) can be an excellent accompanying concept in the therapy or rehabilitation of these illnesses as well as in aftercare, including cancer diseases, especially in health resort medicine. The therapeutic basics needs to be provided by studies based on the current criteria of evidence-based medicine, which have to be carried out in Central European forests and under the appropriate conditions. This opens up a new exciting and comprehensive scientific field.

We can be glad that forest therapy has found its way from Asia to the western world, and we hope that as many people as possible will be able to benefit from it based on the knowledge available to date and in the future.

Index

© Springer-Verlag GmbH Germany, part of Springer Nature 2022
A. Schuh, G. Immich, *Forest Therapy - The Potential of the Forest for Your Health*,
https://doi.org/10.1007/978-3-662-64280-1

Printed in the United States
by Baker & Taylor Publisher Services